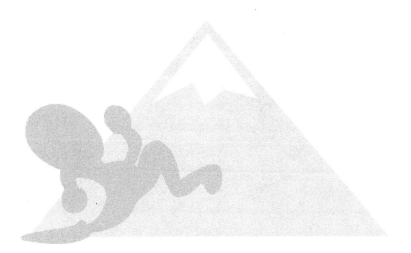

Alpine Weight Loss Secrets

by Stefan Aschan

PRAISE FOR THE
ALPINE WEIGHT LOSS SECRETS
TO LOOK YOUNGER NATURALLY

"I can assure you as a physician that following *The Alpine Weight Loss Secrets* will change your vitality and physique in multiple ways. Stefan Aschan, one of New York City's most respected personal trainers, has a creative, astute and highly entertaining approach to diet and exercise. Follow his advice carefully and the results will be wunderbar."

Stuart Fischer,
MD, author of the *Park Avenue Diet*

"This is a terrific book, loaded with practical, proven methods to lose weight, feel great and enjoy unlimited energy."

Brian Tracey,
Author of the *Goals* and *No Excuses!: The Power of Self-Discipline*

"Several years ago, Stefan Aschan was transplanted from an Alpine village to metropolitan New York. Once he recovered from culture shock, he noticed the plethora of obese people in the big city. As a result, he wrote *Alpine Weight Loss Secrets* in an attempt to coach his new countrymen and countrywomen to adopt sensible eating habits, substituting "empty calories" for "quality calories". The result is a collection of practical suggestions for weight loss that makes sense, that guarantees delightful reading, and may save the life of some readers along the way."

Stanley Krippner,
Ph.D. Professor of Psychology, Saybrook University

"Thank you for changing my life. Post-menopausal, at 51, I thought all I had to look forward to was a downhill slump of more sagging and drooping. In less than two months your exercises and nutritional recipes have helped me to lose the fat, restore tone and muscle to my body, and have given me more energy than I have had in 20 years. I went from 145 lbs to 125 lbs. My friends tell me I look 35, and I have the energy I had at 20. And my sexual appetite has been rekindled! You are a miracle worker."

Susan Hudson, 51,
Former CEO

"When I initiated Stefan's program, I was concerned that it would have a temporary benefit. This was my experience with all previous "diet" programs I had tried in the past, including the popular reduced carbohydrate methods. What I soon realized was that the nutrition program was not a "diet" at all, but rather functioned as a training program for healthy cooking and eating, one of the core ingredients to healthy living. Through the program I was convincingly familiarized with the benefits of natural foods and principles of nutrition that I would never have explored or learned on my own. The benefits have remained simply because I feel better when I eat this way. This experience has been unlike any other "diet" program I had tried in the past, which ultimately failed because they were based on applying restrictions to what I really wanted to do which was to enjoy eating! I went from 30% to 22% body fat, lost 20 lbs as I went from 214 lbs to 194 lbs, and changed my hip measurements from 40.5 inches to 35.5 inches and my waist measurement from 40 inches to 36 inches. And this is really just the beginning. Through my experience with his program, I do not feel restricted but rather feel that I have been opened up to a whole new world of food and gained a tremendous knowledge, which will stay with me for the rest of my life. And even better, I enjoy eating!"

Andrew J. Fishman, 42,
MD, New York University School of Medicine

For more praise visit
www.AlpineWeightLossSecrets.com

COMMON WEIGHT LOSS AND YOUNGEVITY PROBLEMS

Everybody is different. Not just their external body, but also the internal body at the cellular level. Whatever your body type, body concerns, or obstacles to implementation, there is help. Here's what Stefan recommends for these common problems:

Problem 1 – Bulging belly
Solution: Analyze if there might be more than just fat pushing your belly out. And discover how you can flatten your belly with food and one simple activation.

Problem 2 – Hunched-over posture
Solution: Balance your muscular system. Learn the secret concept that few back doctors know.

Problem 3 – A jiggly stomach
Solution: Follow the the Mountain Program to burn not just epidermal body fat but inner organ fat, too.

Problem 4 – A saggy, baggy, wrinkling body
Solution: Use the primal movement patterns that work your body in 3-dimensional ways. They can strengthen, tone, and lift your arms and butt too.

Problem 5 – Lack of energy
Solution: Eat as close as possible to the earth. Discover the foods that are most beneficial for your metabolic function in categories 1 and 2, and damaging for you in category 3.

Problem 6 – Feeling burned out and bored
Solution: Redirect your focus with 7 key questions—they can be your lifesaver.

Problem 7 – Lack of strength and endurance
Solution: The 3R2S system. Discover how it works and how to implement it.

ALPINE
WEIGHT LOSS
SECRETS

THE MOST AMAZING FREE GIFT EVER

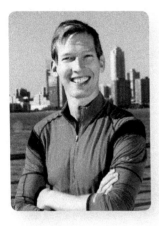

Stefan is offering an incredible opportunity for you to experience first-hand why he is known as Europe's Premier Youngevity Coach.

Since he understands that support is a critical component to success, Stefan will give you on-line support solutions valued at $70, for FREE.

You'll receive the **Longevity Strength Program** workouts to follow at home, outside, or anywhere you like, his Back to Balance Flexibility Program, and access to instructional videos which supplement the program.

Don't miss his continuing updates and smart solutions for weight loss, how to look naturally younger and how to achieve longevity, either!

TO ACTIVATE YOUR MOST INCREDIBLE FREE

GIFT EVER, go to

www.AlpineWeightLossSecrets.com/BookBonusLogIn.html

and access your free gift.

ALPINE
WEIGHT LOSS
SECRETS

ALPINE WEIGHT LOSS SECRETS

The natural way to look and feel 5, 10, or even 20 years younger

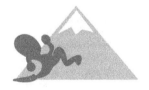

By Stefan Aschan

Europe's Premier Youngevity Coach

Alpine Weight Loss Secrets

Copyright © 2010, Stefan Aschan
First Printing, January 2011
CreateSpace Publishing

Cover & book design: Sylvia Hanousek, www.jobgrafik.at
Editor: Stephanie Young
Photography: Kristina Nazarevskaia www.knstudios.com, Chris Fanning www.chrisfannig.com

Strength 123 Inc.
New York, NY, 10065

1 212 750 3696
info@stefanaschan.com
www.stefanaschan.com
Printed in the United States of America
ISBN-10: 145285792X
EAN-13: 978-1452857923
Strength 123 Inc.

Warning – Disclaimer
The workouts and other health-related activities described in this book were developed by the author and are to be used as an adjunct to improved strengthening, conditioning, health, and fitness. These programs may not be appropriate for everyone. All individuals, especially those who suffer from any disease or are recovering from any injury, should consult their physicians regarding the advisability of undertaking any of the activities suggested in these programs. The author has been tested and researched in the science behind his programs. However, he is neither responsible nor liable for any harm or injury resulting from this program or the use of the exercises or exercise devices described herein.

Attention: Corporations
This book is available at quantity discounts with bulk purchase for educational, business, or sales promotion use. For information, please write to: Special Sales Department, Strength 123 Inc., 791 Lexington Ave, Suite 2R, New York, NY 10065

Acknowledgments

I would like to thank the many individuals who have made this project possible and supported, encouraged, and motivated me to keep going:

My parents, who moved to the tiny village of Streifing from Vienna, Austria.

Esther Diharangirei, my second mother, who pushed, encouraged, and motivated me to go to New York. Without her, this book would not be in your hands.

Karolina Kobetitsch, who said the right things at the right time and provided a different kind of opinion.

Lorna Zawacki for her valuable professional input, feedback, and advice to keep the program simple.

Lesley Friedman, Eunice Valdivia, Kristina Nazarevskaia, Sylvia Hanousek, Jake McDonald, and Konstantine Karides, who kept placing professional decisions in the right perspective.

Special thanks to my editor, Stephanie Young. I thank her from the bottom of my heart for coming on this project and maintaining the right tone in my voice. Without her insight, this book would not be in this current easy-to-read format and perhaps would not have been completed.

My first agents, Sophia Sneider and Judith Ehrlich, for their professional input that made it work and their passion to see it succeed.

My second agent, Karen Ganz Zahler. Without her, this project would have come to a halt at a critical time.

To all my colleagues who provided education that was applied and used to transform my clients into young, energy abundant, and pain-free individuals.

And to all my clients who have helped to form the information in one way or the other. Without you the program would not be in its current form.

This book was an expedition—or rather, a trip to the Alps. There are many ways to reach the peak of a mountain, but stick-to-it-ness is the secret to your success. I believe that you will progress within the first week of this program. But your real peaks will be climbed and reached long after these words have been read.

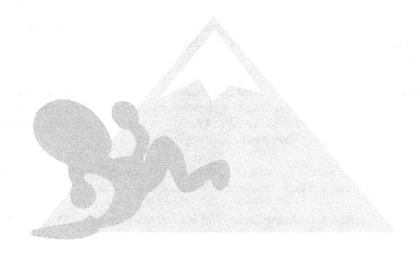

ALPINE
WEIGHT LOSS
SECRETS

TABLE OF CONTENTS

ALPINE
WEIGHT LOSS
SECRETS

ALPINE
WEIGHT LOSS
SECRETS

Alpine Weight Loss Secrets

Introduction

Maybe you don't like what you are seeing and feeling these days. Sagging facial, arm, stomach, and leg muscles; low energy; large belly; hunched-over posture; lost body tone; cellulite; the inability to move; the inability to stay active and independent; and unhappiness over lost youth and opportunities earlier in life are NOT the result of getting older. It is an ugly, slowly growing tumor that spreads and inhibits your capabilities, but you can fight it. You can look and feel your best, enjoy energy, enjoy an attractive, toned body, get back a youthfull attitude about life, experience new joy in your daily life, enjoy active sex, provided you start now.

This book incorporates my knowledge of century-old strategies from the Alpine environment where I grew up, scientific research, and more that 17 years of working as a nutrition and exercise coach. The information is presented in an easy-to-follow and comprehensive program that you can implement as a lifestyle that can and will prevent and reverse the signs of aging, old thinking, an unsexy posture, and the attitude that ages you. We will be looking at weight loss from an Alpine perspective and share strategies that have been naturally followed in a country that was referred to as the "Alpine Power House." A place where you see the 90-year-olds moving, acting, and living like they're 30-somethings. Hip replacements? Knee replacements? Unheard of. There they live happy and contented lives without the aches, pains, diseases, and body shapes that plague so many of us living in large city environments.

After more than 17 years working with individuals to help them lose pounds, shrink inches and body fat, change body appearance and attitude, eliminate aches and pains, teach skills to improve their bodies' capabilities, I finally fine-tuned my approach into a successful program that can and has been implement-ed with at 99.9% success rate. Individuals from all walks of life have profited from this program, including the mother of three whose children moved out, the retired CEO from a Fortune 500 company, the recently divorced secretary trying to find herself again, and models getting ready for photo shoots. The program has also helped young women who were sick and tired of gimmicks and fad diets. I am proud to say that they consistently have left my sessions with great results after implementing my personalized strategies and advice.

By following my program, thinking approach, and strategies, you can achieve and maintain a pain-free body that is agile, toned, and in shape; capable of maintaining balance and staying flexible; and has abundant energy. Your re-claimed health will be reflected in your glowing skin (glowing like the moon in a mountain lake), flat stomach, elastic skin, and muscles like a 25-year-old. Even better, your attitude will improve to the point that you will go out and try one thing that scares you each month—like changing your relationship, finding a new adventure, trying a new cognitive strategy to feel happy and energized again, or starting to date and have sex again after a breakup.

Wait, did I mention that weight will be lost? It will, and you better believe it. You don't have to go under the knife, go for Botox, or resort to liposuction. Even if you do, you still need to stay active to stay independent and strong for the years to come. The information shared in this book is a basic and familiar anthropological truth for how to look and feel younger naturally with Alpine Weight Loss Secrets.

A Lifestyle for Centuries

In the little Alpine village where I grew up and other villages I visited, we ate with gusto—no diets for us. But unlike most people, individuals in Alpine environ-ments tend to eat foods that are close to the earth. "Going to the gym" is not a phrase that is commonly used. Instead, people say, "Let's go for a walk, a hike, a run, or a bike ride." People enjoy each other's company while staying active. The result is a complete package of health, longevity, and youngevity; clear-headedness; and strong, lean, energized bodies. In my Alpine village, people in their 70s look and act 20 or 30 years younger because they are fit, nourished, and active. And, oh boy, can they run after you when you have done something wrong (something I experienced more then once as a teenager!)

This lifestyle approach is instilled in us as very young children. In Alpine environments, activities are an integral part of a daily schedule. It might be just walking to the next village or to the store to buy some food. Why take the car for such a short errand? It is an activity that we enjoy doing because we have been taught to enjoy the journey. My father used to send me to the farm next door (4 miles away) to buy eggs, bread, and beer on the weekends. We would bike to the next village to visit our friends, despite the steep hills between us. Breathing the late summer air, smelling the freshly cut fields, and feeling the warm pockets of wind as you went from one valley to the next were all part of the journey. The experience refreshed the mind. Snowstorm? No problem—the drifts made the journey more interesting. We had fun and did not think it was special then. It was that was normal to us. Being in the moment made us clearheaded ᵃᵈ at our destination.

We achieved this by living with the environment rather than in the environment. Many times we would ask ourselves, "What can I do next? What else can I explore right now? How does this taste? Do I want to do this?"

As I recount my own stories from growing up and combine them with scientific research and years of experience changing my clients' bodies, health, and lives, I lay out a path for you to follow. I take readers through a full program that does not go by day or by phase, but by strategy. We are living in a very busy environment. Sometimes our priorities can change from one day to the next. Would it be best to implement the program from chapter 1 to chapter 11? Yes, but you also can turn to any chapter and start implementing the strategies. You can start with chapter 10 and move to chapter 2. The results will be the same. But for the best results, I provide you with a cohesive approach, organized in the progression in which the book is written.

Here is what you will learn:

Change your mind, change your body: Changing your body starts with your mental muscle. Learn how to flex your mental muscle by following my simple worksheet.

Lighten your metabolism: A calorie is not just a calorie. Chocolate and carrots are not the same. Both affect your system. What is the difference? Might light have an impact? Learn why the glycemic index is misguided, and what you need to watch out for while you implement the forward-thinking research from Germany and Japan that you won't hear about in the States.

Alpine eating – choose tomatoes not potatoes: There are always better decisions you can make when it comes to one food over another. Which is the better choice and what Alpine foods can be eaten to change and maintain a youthful body even in your 90s? All right here.

Improve your fat-titude: Trim the fat in your life. This refers to excessive intake and also things that just slow you down. Learn what kind of fat is good and why. Get educated and learn about fats that burn fat and foods that make you fat.

Instant anti-ager – your posture: Faulty posture does not look good on a teenager and definitely not on an adult of any age in revealing clothes. There are three simple tricks that you can do to improve your posture; these are the basic foundation of any scientific exercise program.

The joy of movement: Too many times have I heard someone say "I hate to exercise." What a shame. Don't blame yourself. One of the first strategies to staying active is to find the activity that you love. And not hate. And this might mean not going to the gym. Discover the other options you have and the strategies that my fellow Alpine villagers have been using to discover joy and form a supportive community.

Train yourself "Jung" (young). Stop sitting around. The more you sit, the weaker you become. In my village, simple everyday strategies are used to stay agile and young. Ditch your old habits with fun, easy-to-remember moves that have been used for centuries in Alpine communities. Of course, I will give you the latest research to back up this approach.

A flat belly – "Schnell" (fast) : Occasional overeating can happen—at big festivals, family gatherings, and the like. But have you over-eaten your entire life? Turn this around fast: *The 2-day Alpine Cleansing Cure* will help give you a flat belly schnell [fast].

The joy of living: Life doesn't end when you are 40, 50, or 60. It begins. Ask yourself these 7 questions that will help you change yourself and provide direction for what you want to be doing next.

Eat yourself thin: Cook and eat. That's my philosophy. But not just any food and not just any cooking technique. Cook the Hudry Wusch way to save time and money. Breakfast, lunch, and dinner prepared according to this new cooking method will leave you satisfied and nourished. You will never return to your old way of cooking.

Stay young for a lifetime: These three ladies, Margarita, Vikki, and Casey have done it. How? Read about their challenges, obstacles, and the approach that worked for them. Pick up one or two things that will work for you.

Now I have a few stories to tell, a lot of strategies to share, and a lot of knowledge to pass on. And I will make you laugh at the same time. I will be driving home basic philosophies and concepts of Alpine living. If you have been looking for a diet book, this is not the right book. If you are looking to lose weight fast and gain it back, this book isn't for you. But if you are looking for change in your thinking and cognitive process of making decisions; strategies that are easy to implement; and for a fun read that provides education and insight about a successful weight loss program that was influenced by strategies learned in my Alpine upbringing, this book is for you. Learning and changing to be a different person and improve your appearance is like preparing for an exciting journey—it's a step-by-step process.

Let's go and let the Alpine advantage begin.

ALPINE
WEIGHT LOSS
SECRETS

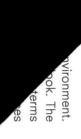

Chapter 1

CHANGE YOUR MIND, CHANGE YOUR BODY

The Choice Is Yours

I love being an adopted European. The opportunities and possibilities that the United States has to offer are endless. Coming from another country can make you feel like an outsider at times, and yet it is up to you to make the change and see situations in various lights. For example, my tendency is always to look at the bright side, and to me, the glass is always half full—not half empty. How we perceive half a glass of water is totally up to us.

Every perception you have is somewhat influenced by the way you were brought up—by mother, father, education, belief system, country, and culture. All these factors have consciously or subconsciously conditioned how your brain is wired.

Look briefly into your decision-making skills when it comes to food choice. Parents can do more damage than good when it comes to this skill. Were you rewarded with food like sweets (perhaps other foods) when you were a child? Years later, long an adult, you may find yourself digging into dessert to reward yourself for getting through a bad day or to celebrate success. Patterns that are set in childhood can influence you today and determine your success in many areas and in any weight loss program.

And how does education fit in? Research has shown that those with higher educational levels make better nutritional choices.

Could religion influence you as well? Yes, just think about kosher food. Kosher is ranked above organic food for its purity, although organic has wider nutritional benefits. The solution? Perhaps kosher organic food?

Growing up in a European country, we are taught the ways of our

country's traditions and eating culture. I was raised in an Alpine ɛ
This conditioned my overall physiology, psychology, palate, and ou
desire to be as close to nature as possible is ingrained in us. Not just in
of activities but also in terms of foods. Today when I see the food cho:
people make in restaurants, the supermarket, or other venues, I can only shak.
my head in disbelief. You also might have seen someone choose Diet Coke for
breakfast! This may be the norm for some, but the first time I saw this, it turned
my stomach. What can I say? We Alpine folks enjoy sitting for a little while in
the morning, enjoying our tea, perhaps a little dark bread with homemade jam,
muesli, or a soft-boiled egg.

Does that mean you are out of luck if your background gave you habits
that are not the best to support a youthful lifestyle? Not at all. But understanding
your underlying belief system can help you understand why you make the same
choices over and over again. Why, for example, you eat sweets after a workout.

Your mental attitude also has a huge impact. How many times have you
said, "I can't"? Yet when you wanted to achieve a goal, you did it. To change
your attitude from I can't to I can, your motivation can come from an unexpected
place. It can even arise from a disturbing realization.

That is exactly what happened to my client Cathy. She is in her 40s and
signed up for checkup and a revamp of her program. After her measurements
were taken, we found that at 5 feet 4 inches and 141 pounds, her percentage of
body fat was 36%, which placed her in the obese category. She was shocked.
Her last checkup with her doctor revealed that she had good cholesterol, and
her cardiovascular system and her digestion were healthy. Yet to truly be healthy,
her body fat percentage should have been between 31% and 21%, and her
weight between 130 pounds and 114 pounds.

Tears rolled down her cheeks as she repeatedly asked, "How did I let it
get this way?" She was at rock bottom but also clearly saw the path that had
led her to this point.

"Are you ready to make a decision that will change your body, your
attitude, and your life?" I asked her after comforting her. She nodded. "Can
you see yourself thinner, younger, happier, and more energetic?" I continued,
"Have you made the decision that you do not want to be here, in this place
of unhappiness and body despair?" She nodded. "If you ever think you cannot do anything or you are too tired or do not have time, think about today's
conversation. Use your clear vision of what you want to become and stay
motivated. Maintain this state of focus and be conscious of your actions
and where you will end up by following them." She started right then and
there. Six months later she had lost 24 pounds and her percentage of body
fat dropped to 21.3%. She went from 141 pounds to 114 pounds. But most
important, she went from I can't to I can.

She flexed her mental muscle, and she was in charge. She made the
decisions that were right for her, starting with that first decision to change.

Flexing Your Mental Muscle

My program will help you to analyze and change your current decision-making process so you make better, clearheaded, more informed choices. This plan will help you rewire your brain with new and better connections. We are not just talking about your decisions about food or how you execute movements. This program will show you how to reprogram how you think about food and activity. **Focus your mind, flex your mental muscle, and the rest will follow.**

How do you flex your mental muscle? It is different for everyone, but one way that many of my clients find helpful is to hit the "pause" button. Think of your life as a series of choices or decisions. At any time—in the next moment, the next hour, the next week—you could choose to stop, to slow down, and to be still for a few seconds. Pausing creates a momentary contrast between your usual response and the choice to make a change. It is the difference between your default mode of distraction and being truly present and conscious of your choices. Just stop, breathe deeply, and choose new. You can use this technique when facing any choice—from whether to eat a piece of candy to whether to explore changing jobs.

The Key Is Finding an Easy Entry Point. Have you ever told yourself that if you would just get back on your daily workout schedule or start a healthy eating plan, the rest of your life would fall back in place? This is true. But that is way too hard. Fixing any one of those problems is just too big. So go for something easier; instead of a whole exercise regimen, do modified push-ups or an abdominal activation morning, noon, and night. You can do it on the floor—any floor—and it takes just 30 seconds. The act of doing one single activity (versus starting a whole new workout) is easy to do. It restarts the momentum of your self-discipline after just a few days.

Warning: You Need to Give up Perfectionism in Order to Get Anywhere. If you are aiming for perfection, you are never going to get yourself to do what you need to do. No one is perfect, and if you tell yourself you need to be perfect, then everything is too hard to start. Remember that the point is not to create additional pressure but to create pleasure. This is the pleasure of accomplishing a goal and sticking to a decision.

Flexing Your Mental Muscle Is All About Believing in Yourself. Take, for example, the person who stops going to group classes for a month. If you think of yourself as someone who enjoys exercising with a group, you are more likely to start going again than if you think of yourself as someone who only works out alone. And this is true in a more broad sense: if you think of yourself as someone with a lot of self-discipline then when you are not exhibiting self-discipline, you expect to start using it again, and you do. Self-discipline is like a muscle, so you need to work it regularly to strengthen it, and part of practicing it is telling yourself that you are a person who has self-control over your own choices.

1
2
3
4
5
6
7
8
9
10
11

MENTAL MUSCLE 101

Flexing Your Mental Muscle Involves Small Things Paving the Way for Very Big Things.

Choosing to take control of how you eat, what you eat, and why you work out puts you in the driver's seat. My advice is to start small because self-discipline snowballs; if you can work hard to have self-discipline in one small area, you create self-discipline almost effortlessly in other areas.

Debbie, one of my first clients, found great success using this approach to bring focus back to her diet. After consulting her food log, we discovered that she used high-calorie foods like mac and cheese at lunch as a reward for accomplishing her morning tasks. This made her tired and mentally sluggish all afternoon. The fix involved suggesting that she should eat warm, broth-based soups as a first course for lunch, and then decide what to eat. The warm soup comforted her and made her feel full so she was less inclined to indulge in the high-calorie entrees. Within a week, she noticed how much more energy she had in the afternoons and she stopped skipping her workout sessions. The simple change at lunchtime gave her the momentum to focus on two other areas that needed improvement: her work and her workout program.

Throughout this book you will encounter worksheets on flexing your mental muscle. Work with me. We are on a journey together, and I am thrilled to help you reach your goal of finding a different lifestyle. Keep a pen handy and fill out the worksheets as you read this book.

Worksheet 1

If you want to improve yourself you need to raise your current standards.
In the lines below, fill in your current standard—use your health, weight,
or activity level. Then raise your standard. Write what you will accomplish.

Current standard for maintaining health:

....

....

New standard for maintaining health:

....

....

Current standard for maintaining weight:

....

....

New standard for maintaining weight:

....

....

Current standard for maintaining activity:

....

....

New standard for maintaining activity:

....

....

Worksheet 2

Next, answer the following: "Why do I want to do this?" Goals are great to have. But without the why behind the what, you will not succeed in the long term. Without the why that is right for you, you will not have an emotional connection that you can reach for to keep going when the going gets rough. Without an emotional connection to your goal, any objective, no matter how good it sounds on paper, does not make sense because you do not know the why.

Take Anna, another client. At 40 years old, she is in a long-term relationship, with no children, and works more than 70 hours a week. In short, she has very little time. Her dream body is something out of a Victoria's Secret catalog. She always mentioned that this is what she aspired to look like. When I asked her why, she explained, "I want to feel comfortable in a bikini on vacation in Italy." With that clear focus and resolve in mind, she went from 139 pounds to 112 lbs. in 12 weeks. Her goal related to her life and not some fantasy. It gave her reason to stay focused. Now it is your turn.

Why do I want to accomplish my new standards?

....

....

....

....

....

....

....

....

....

....

ALPINE
WEIGHT LOSS
SECRETS

Worksheet 3

Your simple entry point! Use common sense. What can you do right now to get started and stick with it for 7 days? Vowing to drink more water? Halve the usual number of soft drinks you currently drink? Not skipping scheduled workouts for a week? Packing a lunch from home? Proving to yourself that you can decide to change and stay with that change is how you start flexing your mental muscle right now. Start your success and record your personal entry point right here.

My personal starting point:

....

....

....

....

....

....

....

....

....

....

....

....

....

| 1 |
| 2 |
| 3 |
| 4 |
| 5 |
| 6 |
| 7 |
| 8 |
| 9 |
| 10 |
| 11 |

These lists will guide you through the program. Keep them at hand. Tape them on your fridge or put them in your Blackberry or cell phone to remind yourself of what you have decided. You can accomplish big results with small steps.

Get It Done! 6 Ways to Flex Your Mental Muscle Today

❶ **Pinpoint your feelings.** There are many emotions that you have to deal with, but the number differs by gender. It has been said that men describe about 8 emotions, but women, about 32. You have to acknowledge and recognize your feelings to work with them. Start a journal with emotional categories such as fear, rejection, worry, helplessness, frustration, depression, boredom, anger, anxiety, etc. Identify the emotions that start a chain of destructive behavior in you. Note when they strike (when you are tired, hungry, or stressed) so you can learn your patterns.

❷ **Control your emotions.** As soon as you know why you feel a particular emotion in a given situation, you can start to control the emotion. You can do this in 3 seconds. Ask yourself: Is it really as bad as I think it is? Think: Am I hoping for better results so I do not have to feel that emotion? Try thinking about a goal that you hope to accomplish. Now think about the same goal and expect it to happen. Don't you feel a difference in the way it empowers you? Expect that you will do well. Raise your bar and perform accordingly. And remember, to hope is not the approach to use to get something done. Expect it to happen.

❸ **Know your stumbling blocks.** Know upfront the obstacles that keep you falling off the goal-accomplishment wagon. If you know them ahead of time, you can work to avoid them.

❹ **Start acting.** This does not have to be physical. It can be a notion that this is going to bring you closer to why you want to accomplish your goal.

❺ **Give yourself the right to change.** Yes, making the commitment to exercise consistently and go to the farmer's market instead of the corner store takes time. But you are not being selfish; you are investing in yourself. You have the right to look good, have energy, and feel good about yourself.

❻ **Stop the blame game and get out of your own way.** You have every right to accomplish your goals. If you're honest, you'll realize that most of the time you are the one who is holding yourself back. Yes, I have heard about your family emergencies, your professional pressure, or the stresses of your life. Yet when is your time for you? When is your time to relax or your time to work out? Analyze how much time you carve out for yourself to work on your goals.

You can have many goals, such as financial independence, changing your body's appearance and health, spending more time with friends or family, becoming more effective with daily tasks... the list goes on. Yet your success starts with your first step. What is your first step—for you—going to be today? **Start flexing your mental muscle TODAY.**

Chapter 2

"LIGHTEN" YOUR METABOLISM

Growing up in an Alpine environment shaped how I eat. Fresh vegetables, fruit, and herbs came from our back garden or from the neighboring farmer's fields. As kids, we were delighted to discover an edible green growing on the side of a dirt road or field. In our tiny village of 20 houses and 3 farms, such food information was shared. If a neighbor thought one of us Aschans was looking too pale, which was attributed to iron deficiency, you can be sure that somehow nettles and dandelions found their way into our house and into our salads. Whether you liked it or not, there was never an argument about eating it. There was no choice. As children, we followed the trustworthy advice of the healthy, slim, and wise elders. (But do you really think we did it without kicking and screaming? Of course not.)

Fast forward 27 years, when I found myself in the United States, where this local, fresh-from-the-fields information and basic green knowledge was replaced with generalized (and often erroneous) information from television, newspapers, and the Internet. The exciting discovery was not that the chives were sprouting in the nearby woods but that a celebrity somewhere on the planet had lost weight with some new faddish plan.

We tend to swallow this information without considering our specific individual needs or how it suits our living environment or life cycle. We cannot trust our instincts anymore as we are so far removed from the earth. Global food shipping means we do not eat according to the season; we can defy the rhythms of day and night thanks to electricity and distractions such as TV and the Internet. Our clearheadedness has been anesthetized. Supermarket specials to buy 2 and get 1 free determine our nutritional intake, and weekend marathons of TV specials dictate our activity levels.

I know because this happened to me, but I did not know it at the time. Changes in food and culture from one continent and environment (Austrian,

Alpine) to another (New York City, urban) affected me within weeks. Upon arriving in New York City, I found success, thanks to my teaching style, at the same gyms where Arnold Schwarzenegger used to train. Pretty soon everyone taking my classes started calling me "Little Arnold." My classes were packed and more private clients signed up to work with my fitness program. No one had ever seen anybody train clients the way we did back home, so people kept coming up to me during sessions to ask for my card. My business was on a roll.

But also something was definitely wrong. It did not happen overnight. A new-to-me tiredness set in. Of course, there was a lot of wear and tear on my body from teaching many hours a week, but I had been this intensely physical my entire life. Sleeping even more hours than I was used to did not leave me refreshed. Then a European friend, who had had similar problems when she moved to the States, asked me a simple question: "What are you eating?"

During my first months in New York, I ate like an American; I ate whatever was served and finished everything on my plate. Like a native, I grabbed food from a corner deli because it was quick, efficient, and inexpensive. Eating processed food loaded with sugars, fats, preservatives, and food coloring was taking a toll on me, and my body paid the price. My body was not suffering from a lack of food—my body was suffering from lack of nutrition. That was the last time I ate like an American, believe me!

If you have been eating mostly processed foods, fried foods, or low quality produce, your body may be suffering from their damaging effects, including weight gain, digestive issues like bloating, looking older than you really are, and other serious health problems. You can change all that and supercharge your metabolism by changing the quality of the food you eat.

Hubert, 39 years old, one of my clients, experiences similar body fat and weight issues when he travels between Europe (Germany and Austria) and the United States (New York). Whenever I see him in New York after a business trip abroad, I always take measurements. That is when he confesses to his indulgence in good food and going out in Europe. Yet, surprisingly, his body fat measurements, over and over again, reveal a lower percentage of body fat when returning from a stay in Europe versus staying for weeks in the United States. This is why I began questioning the quality of the European food system and comparing it to the American food system. I also looked at typical weight loss/maintenance supported by each system.

Your Metabolism, Only Better!

People often think that the metabolism is simply how we burn off food, but it is actually the sum of all the chemical processes, both good and bad, that occur at the cellular level. For optimal energy, health, and youngevity, all those functions and systems need to be working efficiently and in unison. That is when you lose weight, burn off the excess organ fat, and rejuvenate your skin. You

ALPINE
WEIGHT LOSS
SECRETS

also reduce your risk of cancer, cardiovascular disease, high blood pressure, high cholesterol, diabetes, osteoarthritis, rheumatoid arthritis, and inflammation, as well as a myriad other health concerns.

Most popular diet books and even many scientific studies that compare high-carbohydrate or low-fat or high-protein eating plans usually come down to watching your calorie intake. But no one seems to be making what is the most critical distinction—the difference between quality foods such as fresh, organic, and processed foods (produce, meat, and poultry) that have been produced without pesticides, herbicides, antibiotics, and other chemicals. It is not surprising that people who lose lots of weight often regain it (and more) pretty quickly. They have not learned to nourish and satisfy their bodies.

Alpine Secret: Eat Quality Calories

Not all calories are alike. And a quality calorie is more than just a calorie. A fresh, organic apple and a candy bar may both have 90 calories, but there is a world of difference in how those calories interact with your body. That organic apple is packed with nutrients, enzymes, vitamins, and trace minerals (among other things) that fuel your metabolic functions and give you energy. Quality calories stimulate your taste buds so that your stomach registers a sense of fullness and satisfaction. You can actually eat more of these quality calories because the body is utilizing the nutrition very efficiently.

The calories from that candy bar slow down your metabolism, weaken your immune system, and contribute to toxicity buildup. They also take nutrients out of your body rather than putting them in. Such empty calories age your body because they tax your digestive, immune, cardiovascular, and other systems. Those calories make you feel bloated and lethargic. If you eat poorly, you do not have energy, and when you start a weight loss and exercise program, energy is what you need. When you are constantly looking for more food to boost your energy levels, you keep eating. It is why you are still hungry even an hour after a big meal. Many people tell me, "I eat very little, but I still gain weight." If this is the case you need to look at the quality of your calories and make adjustments.

Since quality calorie foods do not have labels proclaiming them as such (at least not yet!), here is how to find them:

Eat More Sunshine

Quality calories are ones found in live food. Foods from Alpine fields or meat that was grass fed on Alpine meadows are not the same as frozen foods or meat from agricultural farms. Make the distinction between live and dead food. You are a living organism and the same should be true of the food you eat. Why eat something that has no vital energy? Recognize that when manufacturers process, package, and strip food of nutrients in an effort to extend shelf life, they are often turning live food into empty calories and dead food. That is really bad news for your metabolism. Do you think there is anything that is naturally nutritious in white bread, canned vegetables, or that fried chicken? I did not think so.

One important way to gauge the vitality of food is the light it emits. For nearly 40 years, Fritz-Albert Popp, a renowned German biophysicist, has been investigating the role light plays in living organisms, especially the human body. We all know that plants are nourished from sunlight. Photosynthesis in plants converts the electromagnetic energy of sunlight into nourishment in the form of biological energy. Photons, the basic unit of light, transfer their energy to seal oxygen and water molecules into glucose, which becomes a food source. Animals and humans, who live directly or indirectly from plants, break open glucose bonds, converting the constituents into carbon dioxide and water, the raw materials for plants to make more food. But that is not all.

What is left is the light energy. Until Popp began his research, it was not completely understood how our bodies use that light. He discovered that this dynamic web of light, which is constantly released and absorbed by our DNA, is the principle regulating mechanism for all life processes. Digest that for a moment: Light is the principle regulating mechanism for all life processes. Popp called these emissions biophotons, which are essentially electromagnetic waves stored in cells' DNA. Biophotons also serve as an organism's main communications network, chemically connecting its cells, tissues, and organs.

A few years ago, Popp, who is highly regarded throughout much of Europe and Russia, was asked to assess the difference between organic food and typical supermarket fare. Using specially constructed equipment to photograph and measure the light emissions, he found that conventional produce, frozen vegetables, eggs, and chicken had very faint emissions, which meant they had little light storage capacity. Preservatives, additives, radiation, long-term storage, pasteurization, canning, freezing, and drying can kill nutrients and the light storage in food.

On the other hand, Popp found that local organic foods had the same type of coherent and consistent light he found in healthy cells. His conclusion: when you eat a local, organic tomato, you absorb and distribute its life-giving light and reinforce your body's highly calibrated regulatory and communication systems, generating renewal at a cellular level.

Worksheet 4

Lighten up your food intake! How much light food do you eat in one day? By that I mean food that is free of preservatives, additives, and radiation and that has not been stored long term, pasteurized, canned, frozen, or dried. Write down the foods you eat on a typical day and draw a "sun" sign next to each "live" item; food that also comes from a local possible organic source (within 30 miles) also merits a sun sign. Look at your list. The goal is to eat more light daily!

Your one-day food intake:

....

....

....

....

....

....

....

....

....

....

....

....

....

....

....

1
2
3
4
5
6
7
8
9
10
11

Eat Your Enzymes

Energy is obviously necessary to the existence of each living cell, but enzymes are important too. Enzymes are proteins that act as catalysts in making all metabolic functions possible. If the right enzymes are not present, those chemical reactions become disorganized and uncontrolled. So enzyme deficiency can have a devastating effect on your body.

Our cells take energy from three main macronutrients—carbohydrates, protein, and fats. Oxygen reacts with those components in chemical reactions inside the cells, breaking these macronutrients into the micro-nutrients (amino acids, glucose, and fatty acids), releasing energy called adenosine triphosphate or ATP, the universal energy currency for your metabolism. The amount of energy released through oxidation (or, this reaction with oxygen) is measured in calories.

Without constantly renewing the supply of nutrients through your diet, your cells cannot function properly. There are digestive, metabolic, and food enzymes, and when your body does not get enough live enzymes from your food, your pancreas, stomach, and small intestine must work that much harder to produce more digestive enzymes to metabolize what you eat. That is very tax-ing! The less you make your body work, the better.

Live enzymes are derived from foods consumed in their natural, uncooked state. When food is cooked to 118° F, most live enzymes are destroyed. So are many of the vitamins. For example, various estimates are that 50% of B vitamins, 97% of folic acid, and up to 80% of vitamin C are lost through cooking. It is the same for processed foods that have been heated to extend their shelf life. So most of us are getting between 15% to 50% of the nutritive value and 0% of the live enzymes from the food we eat every day.

Of course, nobody wants to (or should) eat raw meat or fish (sushi not-withstanding), so you need to get most of these nutrients from eating fresh fruits and raw vegetables. Another source of live enzymes is yogurt and some cheeses such as farmer's cheese, kefir, or quark (a thick, spreadable cheese that is very common in Europe and is similar to cottage cheese. You can buy it at many farmers markets). Some spreadable cheeses also contain live enzymes; read the ingredients and look for the friendly bacteria.

Karen, a 43-year-old mother of one, started my program because she had to lose the baby weight. It just was not happening, and it had been 10-plus years! She worked in the fashion industry and knew how to be beautiful on the outside. During our interview she revealed that her post-pregnancy food intake was restricted. She kept her energy level up with sugar, Diet Coke, and spinning classes here and there. She did not realize that this diet and haphazard activity schedule affected her appearance, skin tone, and energy. After I educated her about enzymes and sun foods, Karen began incorporating the recommended foods into her diet. She also made a resolution to walk outside daily, even if it was for only 15 minutes, and try to get to spin classes more regularly.

Getting her to cut out the caffeine and sugar was a tough sell, but I kept telling her that she would feel better fast. And she did. By the second week, she saw a huge improvement in her skin, and she was waking up with energy that she only experienced after a sugar, chocolate, or Diet Coke infusion. I have to say, she was not a believer about my promise that this approach would turning back her physical-aging clock. But then the compliments started: colleagues and strangers remarked how refreshed she looked. Today her shopping cart is no longer a guilt cart of guilty pleasures but full of vital energy.

Worksheet 5

Eat more enzymes. Live enzymes are found in foods that are unheated or are not heated above 118° F. Write down the foods you eat for one day. Then place an edelweiss sign next to the item that has its enzymes and vital energy intact. (Do not confuse an enzyme food with a light food. There is a subtle difference; an enzyme food is uncooked and could come from far away. Light foods need to come from local organic sources.)

My raw foods for one day:

....

....

....

....

....

....

....

....

....

....

1
2
3
4
5
6
7
8
9
10
11

Today I live in New York City and have found my little village habits again. It took me some time, but even living in a large city, you can find solutions that will fit your lifestyle. My discovery was the farmers markets dotted around the city. I advise my clients to just go once a week to the markets. They do not have to buy anything at first; I encourage them simply to get reacquainted with seasonal foods, to be in touch with the local providers, and to see the difference between supermarket foods and green, sunlight food. Believe me, you can smell, feel, see, and taste the difference.

Leaving the city to go upstate to a little village called Cold Spring was another discovery. It is a century-old village with history and lots of dirt roads located in the forest. One summer night, my friends and I picked blackberries fresh from the bushes. Our hiking trip was shortened because of our indulgence in the fresh, ripe blackberries. Once again, I discovered dandelions and forest chives growing wild all over the place. If I did not eat them on the spot, they were part of my next meal. Really, there are many ways you can find your "Alpine village" that lightens your metabolism anywhere you go.

8 WAYS TO LIGHTEN YOUR YEARS

Implementation can be challenging; here are 8 simple ways to start. Lighten your years with more enzymes, quality calories, and foods filled with sunlight. You can do it today.

❶ **Eat fresh.** Try to eat something fresh with every meal. Back home we often start a meal with a romaine salad with herbs, tomatoes mixed with oil and vinegar, onion salad, or a shredded carrot salad with raisins, a little oil, and lemon juice.

❷ **Go for greens.** The other way to change and cleanse is with a big green salad with lots of vegetables, such as carrots, broccoli, tomatoes, and radishes, which have a lot of vitamin C (a collagen booster).

❸ **Think before you bite.** Did the vegetable come from a can? Was it transported from thousands of miles away? Grown without pesticides? Cooked until unidentifiable? Ask yourself this question: Where did this food come from before I bought it? If you don't know, don't buy it. In a restaurant, ask the waiter or find out. Optimally, you should know where your food is coming from.

❹ **Eat sulfur-rich foods.** Alpine folks also eat many sulfur-rich foods such as eggs, onions, and garlic. These act as amino-rich emulsifiers that help with bile production. Again, that means better digestion of fats, weight loss, and a more efficient metabolism. Raw onions in particular nourish the friendly bacteria in your stomach.

ALPINE
WEIGHT LOSS
SECRETS

❺   **Supercharge with sprouts.** Another readily available source of enzymes is vegetable sprouts. Consider that sprouts are all about germination and growth, so it makes sense that they are literally enzyme factories. There are so many mail order sources (just Google organic sprouts) and inexpensive, easy-to-use sprouters (a sunny counter or windowsill will do) to choose from. You can grow anything from wheatgrass to broccoli or radish sprouts and add the crunch of vital enzymes in your salads or sandwiches.

❻   **Add herbs.** Use a few fresh sprigs of herbs such as sage or basil leaves in a dish. Or toss some cilantro or flat leaf parsley into a salad. Those that are organic and grown in your window box or garden are the best source of vital enzymes and light energy.

❼   **Fire up the juicer.** Enjoy a glass or two of fresh carrot and celery juice with a drop of olive oil, which slows down absorption to stabilize insulin. A fresh glass of carrot and parsley juice is like drinking sunshine and pure nutrients. You will read more about the advantages of juicing in my program a little later.

❽   **Go raw.** Instead of cooking your favorite vegetables, try them raw. You will be getting loads of light energy, enzymes, and phytochemicals in the process.

1
2
3
4
5
6
7
8
9
10
11

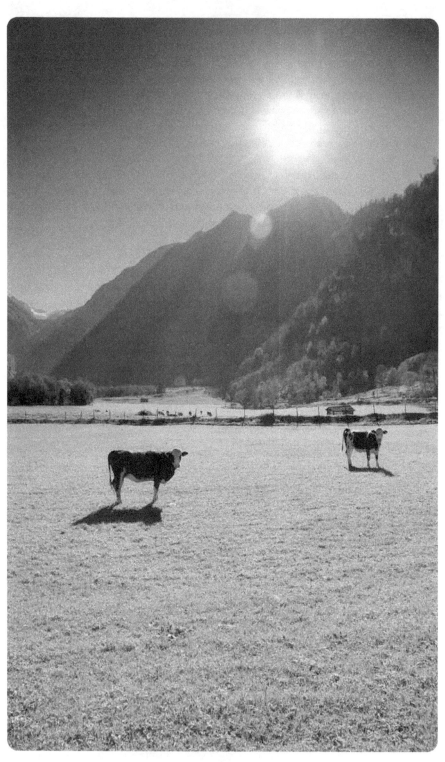

ALPINE
WEIGHT LOSS
SECRETS

Chapter 3

ALPINE EATING: CHOOSE TOMATOES NOT POTATOES

1
2
3
4
5
6
7
8
9
10
11

Travel is a wonderful experience and education at the same time. One of my fondest memories is driving from Vienna to Salzburg and then to Zurich. You are surrounded on all sides by the fresh-air sky and the lushness of green meadows. After a rain, the air is filled with the freshness of mountain air, grass, and flowers. The meadows are dotted with cows, sheep, and horses. But the memory you take away is the clanking of the bells from the milk cows as they walk from one new green spot to the next.

There is another reason that I bring up the cows and lushness of the environment. There are many benefits to be gained from the milk and meat of grass-fed animals. The grass in Alpine meadows contains a special ingredient that has been studied for its anti-cancer and tumor-fighting ability, as well as for its ability to reduce accumulation of abdominal fat. Conjugated linoleic acid (CLA) is the name of this wonder ingredient that helps you burn body stores of fat. An American study of 80 overweight people found that those who took CLA when they dieted and regained the weight when the diet ended put the weight on as 50% muscle and 50% fat. Those who did not take CLA regained the weight at 75% fat and 25% muscle, the usual ratio of weight gain.

According to Michael Pariza, PhD, whose team carried out the study, CLA works by reducing the body's ability to store fat while it promotes the use of stored fat for energy. CLA is a metabolic enhancer, helping convert fat to lean muscle tissue, and grass-fed animals are a key source. When cows are fed grain, a common practice in the States, even as little as two pounds a day, their production of CLA plummets. This may be one reason many Alpine people are so fit and trim even in old age. They receive plenty of CLA through the meat and milk products from Alpine meadow-fed animals.

Foods that support the digestive system also keep older people youthful.

Through the aging process our bodies produce less digestive juices to help break down the food that we eat to nourish our cells, organs, muscles, and skin. There are some specific foods that have traditionally been consumed in my little Alpine village. They are part of the reason why everyone there is so trim and fit. (The other half of the equation is how active they are from sunup to sunset.)

11 Alpine Metabolic Boosters

Try these simple, healthy village youngevity metabolic boosters:

❶   **Power up with peppermint tea.** This minty herb stimulates digestion and cleanses the liver, which is key for fat metabolism. As you age, your digestion is key to youth as it breaks down food into usable components that your cells can use to rejuvenate, rebuild, and maintain.

❷   **Soak the oats.** Muesli! European muesli is raw rolled oats that have been soaked in water, served with yogurt, nuts, lemon juice, and seasonal fruits. Oats don't have to be cooked. Oats turbo-charge your immune system, have more protein than any popular cereal, have a lowering effect on blood sugar, and are high in soluble and insoluble fiber (55% and 45%). Beta-glucan, a polysaccharide, helps lower cholesterol and significantly reduces the risk of cardiovascular disease and stroke. Instant oat packets do not count as they are highly processed and contain sugars.

❸   **Seek out cider.** Alpine folks use a lot of raw apple cider vinegar because it replenishes healthy bacteria in your stomach. Salad dressings are prepared with raw apple cider vinegar. And sometimes, as a refreshment and digestive aid, we enjoy a teaspoon of raw apple cider vinegar in sparkling water before a meal.

❹   **Love the yogurt.** Yogurt is eaten for the same reason. Go for plain and organic. Skip the ones with flavors and fruits on the bottom because they are a sugar fest you do not need. Instead, use fresh seasonal fruits and/or a dollop of raw honey to add texture and additional flavor. There is nothing better than a bowl of homemade strawberry yogurt on a Saturday afternoon!

❺   **Look to lemon juice.** Lemon juice, in particular, aids in digestion and fat breakdown as lemon increases hydrochloric acid production (a digestive juice) and bile production, which is a fat emulsifier. Lemon juice also helps cleanse the liver. The liver is the Grand Central Station of fat conversion. Start your day with this Alpine eye opener: drink one glass of water with the juice of one lemon.

❻   **Spread the Liptauer**. Spice it up. Instead of sugary snacks, we tend to go for metabolic boosters, such as the spices found in Liptauer spread (see recipe on page 175). Liptauer has cayenne pepper and paprika, which are thermogenic or heat-generating spices. Try some on a piece of chewy rye bread. Another village formula: bread with little butter and some fresh chives, which are antibacterial and antifungal. I pick chives all the time when I am hiking and then munch away as I walk. In the spring you can find them in forests. You can often smell them when they are young and it has recently rained.

❼ **Pull out the pumpkin seed oil.** It has been used for centuries in monasteries up in the Alps. Generations ago, the monks discovered the many health benefits of this oil, which is now being reevaluated in the scientific world. Studies have shown that pumpkin seed oil contains more than 60% to 90% unsaturated fatty acids and vitamins and minerals such as A, B1, B2, B6, C, D, E, and K. It has very high levels of antioxidants and polyunsaturated fats, including fatty acids such as palmitic, stearic, linoleic, and oleic acids. This oil is a liver detoxifier and skin rejuvenator and is an important contributor to health because of its B vitamin content.

❽ **Open the sardines.** In Alpine villages, people consume local fish like trout, carp, and salmon trout. These fish are high in omega 3 and omega 6 fatty acids. There are so many benefits for women from these essential fatty acids that books have been written about them. Let's just look at a few of them: building blocks for RNA and DNA; relief from many perimenopausal symptoms; lowered risk of blood clots; relaxation of blood vessels; improved complexion; strengthening of skin, hair, and nails; weight loss, and clearing of such skin conditions as dry skin, acne, and psoriasis. The omegas combat depression and lower the risk of breast cancer. That is the short version. And because cooking fresh fish can smell up the kitchen and a whole one might be too large for one person to eat, consider sardines. Sardines in a can (the only canned food that I promote in this book) are a great snack, easy to prepare, and always available.

❾ **Reach for hearty rye.** If you have ever been to Alpine villages, you know that you can find a large variety of very thick, dense breads. Opt for rye, which has more nutrients than white bread because it is made from whole grain. The fiber content in whole grain is maintained compared to its counterpart of processed flour. The sourdough version (vs. the yeast version) helps to nurture our internal digestive flora or healthy bacteria.

❿ **Grate horseradish.** Puah! You will be laughing when you taste freshly grated horseradish and think about the Alpine weight loss secrets. Then you will start crying as it cleans your sinuses and nose. And later you will experience a great functioning digestion. Horseradish is a digestive stimulant, and it inhibits bacterial infection and increases circulation. This root beats even broccoli, although both belong to the cruciferous family. Research has shown that vegetables belonging to that family have tremendous health benefits and cancer-fighting properties, but did you know that horseradish is one of the richest sources of allyl isothiocyaate, which plays a role in prevention and suppression of tumors and tumor growth? Additionally, there is ten times the amount of glucosinolates in horseradish than in broccoli, according to Dr. Mosbah Kushad, professor at the University of Illinois. Glucosinolates increase the liver's ability to detoxify carcinogens.

16   **Cut the kohlrabi.** What is it? That is the question you will be asked when you offer friends this tasty, crunchy, and easy-to-cut vegetable. Kohlrabi stew was one of the stews Alpine children grew up with. And what child loves vegetables? If, back then, someone would have suggested eating it raw, with a little sprinkle of sea salt, it would have been the Alpine popcorn. Kohlrabi is high in fiber, a good source of vitamin C, an excellent source of potassium, and only 36 calories per cup.

Carrots, beetroot, celery, spinach, parsley, and cucumbers are other items that are typically consumed. These you will encounter again in the chapter, *A Flat Belly – "Schnell" (fast)!* when you learn about the special benefits of those food items and how they benefit your system.

Fresh Air Foods That Can Lose You 30 Pounds

The Alpine foods listed above contribute to maintaining youthful skin, producing abundant energy, and yielding a youthful, healthy body. Introducing these foods into your current nutrition plan will be a good start. Still, how do you accomplish results that you, your colleagues, friends, family, and spouse will see and feel? That you can measure in the circumference of your belly? That you can see in less body weight? This will take a little bit more than just adding 16 foods to your eating plan. Why? Your usual diet might include sugar, caffeine, processed foods, preservatives, and additives.

How can you achieve a weight loss of 30 or more pounds? How can you fit into that dress from 20 years ago? How can you have thinner arms, thinner legs, and a thinner waist again? How can you feel your hips and your ribs again? Or perhaps see a long, slender neckline? This you can accomplish with my Alpine Eating Plan. So many individuals have used my plan to change their appearance, stop the need for their blood pressure medication, and lose the weight once and for all. You can do all this….and not count calories. My experience has shown that women know how to count calories. What they don't know is which foods are rejuvenating, not taxing, and will help them achieve a younger system on a cellular level again.

We are not starting out with counting calories. No. You need to eat. My strategy with this program is to provide you with options. You choose and pick the food items on the list that fit your palate and are easily found in your area so you can stay on the program for the next couple of days.

How to Start the Transformation

The plan calls for eating as close to the earth as possible for the next 14 days. Think fresh, clean, and green. You will want to choose the freshest, cleanest food you can find for yourself—free of preservatives, fillers, dyes, pesticides, and other chemicals that leave your body starving for nutrients.

You need to eat foods high in chemicals from plants that protect cells from oxidative stress, which accelerates aging. These foods are high in conjugated linoleic acid that aids in weight and fat loss; they replenish energy because of their low glycemic load; and they prevent diseases that are common in industrial environments where food has been overly processed and stripped of nutritional value. These are foods filled with light and enzymes; these foods are found in the fields—not in a package or a can. They are Fresh Air Foods.

Fresh Air Foods have only touched fresh air. Specifically, food that has not been packaged, transported, and stored in plastic. I'm talking about vegetables and fruits. Grains, nuts, seeds, fish, and meats are fine in some form of container, as long as there are no additional chemicals added to prolong storage. Choosing these foods is a way of going green from the outside in. This approach not only brings you closer to the earth and natural foods, but it is also good for the planet. It is eco-friendly.

Chemical-free foods keep our drinking water cleaner; remember your body consists of about 90% water. Consuming local foods means less carbon dioxide emissions from large trucks and airplanes that transport food. Thankfully my village was "green" when I was growing up long before there was a green revolution.

Minding Your Menus

Let me tell you this: It starts with you!

If you do not control what you eat, everybody around you will control it for you—from your family, friends, and advertisers to your local supermarket and the nearby fast-food places. What you eat will either energize or deplete your metabolism.

You can make poor food choices, age badly, and destabilize your immune, cardiovascular, hormonal, and other essential systems or you can eat smarter and improve these systems. You can eat to gain weight or lose it. You can limit yourself to a narrow set of food choices or open yourself up to a much broader range of tastes, textures, and satisfying eating experiences. It is really that simple.

How to Use the Fresh Air Food Charts

The best: These are the most important foods; ones that support your metabolic functions, cleansing and rejuvenation, and weight loss efforts.

Good: These are also important nutritional foods for you but not as important as the category above.

Stay away from: These are the foods you should stay away from while improving your decision-making process to achieve weight reduction and age loss. Do not eat them.

When you start with this way of eating, stick to foods from the best and good categories. Foods from the stay away list will slow down your weight loss and anti-aging progress at first. Some of them will be reintroduced when you have completed the first 14 days. Then you can indulge yourself occasionally with items from this list once you have experienced what it feels to have a functioning metabolism and a working digestive system. Stick with it.

Do not stress about all this structured eating. Think about it! If you eat 35 meals per week (5 per day 7 days a week), you can have one that is off track and you will probably be doing better than you were before you began the program. After all, 34 great meals and one not-so-great meal is a good ratio.

Picking the Proper Foods

Focus on balancing your meals among vegetables (fibrous carbohydrates), carbohydrates (starchy carbohydrates), and protein. Use fats with every meal. Opt for Fresh Air Foods that are locally grown and/or organic. Choose meats from grass-fed animals and fish that are not farmed (wild preferred). It would be best to consume the vegetables raw, lightly steamed, or baked. Meats and fish should be grilled or roasted.

For one week focus on using the best foods. For the second week, expand to the good foods. Let's go. Read on and start implementing today. Practice flexing your mental muscle with these foods.

ALPINE
WEIGHT LOSS
SECRETS

THE BEST

VEGETABLES	CARBO-HYDRATES	PROTEIN	FATS
Asparagus	Amaranth	Chicken	Pumpkin Seed Oil
Beets	Barley	Mackerel	Extra Virgin
Bok Choy	Brown Rice	Sardines	Olive Oil
Broccoli	Millet	Wild Salmon	Black Currant
Brussels Sprouts	Oats (groats,	Eggs	Seed Oil
Cabbage	whole, or scotch)		Flaxseed Oil
Carrots	Quinoa	Adzuki Beans	
Cauliflower	Rye	Black Beans	**NUTS / SEEDS**
Daikon	Teff	Garbanzo Beans	Pumpkin Seeds
Dulse	Wild Rice	Lentils	Sunflower Seeds
Garlic		Kidney Beans	Almonds
Green Beans		Pinto Beans	(raw and unsalted)
Green Onions		Red Beans	Flaxseeds
Green Peppers		Romano Beans	(ground)
Kale			
Kelp			
Leeks			
Lentils			
Mung Bean			
Sprouts			
Napa Cabbage			
Onions			
Peppers (red,			
yellow, orange)			
Scallions			
Seaweeds			
Squash			
Turnips			

1
2
3
4
5
6
7
8
9
10
11

GOOD

VEGETABLES	CARBO-HYDRATES	PROTEIN	FATS
Artichokes (cooked)	Arrowroot	Codfish	**NUTS / SEEDS**
Alfalfa Sprouts	Buckwheat (Kasha)	Haddock	Hazelnuts
Bamboo Shoots	Bulgur Wheat (Tabouli)	Halibut	Pecans
Beet Greens	Chick-pea Flour	Herring	Pine Nuts
Celery	(besan, chana,	Salmon	Sesame Seeds
Chives	garbanzo)	Swordfish	Tahini
Collard Greens	Couscous	Trout	
Cucumbers	Spelt Bread	Turkey	
Fava Beans	Whole Wheat	Tuna	
Fennel	Rolled Oats		
Kohlrabi		Seitan	
Lettuces (except Iceberg)	(Breads should not contain processed	Tofu	
Mung Beans	flour, sugar, or	**DAIRY**	
Mustard Greens	yeast. Whole	Butter (very small	
Parsley	grains only.)	amounts)	
Parsnips		Butters (almond,	
Peas (green)		filbert, pecan,	
Radishes		sesame, sun-	
Shallots		flower, and	
Snow Peas		pumpkin only)	
Spinach		Milks made from	
Swiss Chard		brown rice or other	
Tomatoes		grains (watch for	
Turnip Greens		sugar content –	
Water Chestnuts		not sweetened	
Yams		with cane sugar,	
Zucchini		molasses, or su-	
		cranate, etc.)	
		Yogurt (plain,	
		low-fat, or nonfat)	

ALPINE
WEIGHT LOSS
SECRETS

STAY AWAY FROM

VEGETABLES	CARBO-HYDRATES	PROTEIN	FATS
Tomato Juice (heated only)	Miller's Bran	**MEAT/FISH**	**DAIRY**
Watercress	Oat Bran	Perch	Farmer's Cheese
Artichoke Hearts (marinated)	Popcorn	Red Snapper	Feta Cheese
Canned Veg-	Wheat Bran	Sardines (canned)	Quaark Cheese
etables	Wheat Germ	Tuna (canned)	Ricotta Cheese
Celeriac	Basmati White Rice	Bacon	Tofu Cheese
Eggplant	Black or Red Rice	Beef	Amazake
Endive	Bread (made with white flour)	Clams	Cheese (all cheeses)
Escarole	Cereals (refined, dry, or ground whole grain)	Crab	Cottage Cheese
Haricots	Chips (of any kind)	Duck	Cream
Iceberg Lettuce	Corn	Goose	Cream Cheese
Lima Beans	Cornmeal	Ham	Kefir
Mushrooms (ex-cept Shitake)	Cornstarch	Hamburger	Margarine
Navy Beans	Crackers	Hot Dogs	Milk
Northern Beans	Granola	Lamb	Processed Cheeses
Okra	Macaroni	Liver	Soy
Pickled Vegetables	Oatmeal (instant)	Lobster	
Pimentos	Pastas	Luncheon Meats	
Potatoes	Rice Cakes	Mussels	**NUTS**
Potatoes (yellow, sweet)	White Rice	Octopus	Brazil Nuts
Pumpkin	White Wheat Flour	Organ Meats	Cashews
Radicchio	Tempeh	Oysters	Chestnuts
Rhubarb	Yeast	Rabbit	Coconuts & Coconut Oils
Rutabagas		Pickled Herring	Macadamias
Split peas		Pork	Peanut Butter
Wax Beans		Processed Meats	Pistachios
White Beans		Sausages	Walnuts
		Scallops	
		Shellfish	
		Shrimp	
		Smoked Meats	
		Squid	
		Sushi	
		Venison	

1
2
3
4
5
6
7
8
9
10
11

What to do with this list? There is help! That's why you will be provided with recipes and ideas what to do with this program the next 14 days in the *Hudry Wusch Eat Yourself Thin* chapter. Go there now or read on if you are looking for more structure.

Case Study: Erasing Years and Pounds
in a Handful of Days

Andy, a 45-year-old doctor, was disappointed by his previous efforts to lose weight. He was in good shape and worked out with a trainer regularly but had stopped seeing any significant results. When he consulted with me, he was concerned that my program would yield only the temporary results he had experienced with other programs.

His challenge was to keep an open mind and try something new. When he started with my program, he quickly realized that the program was not a diet at all but rather a training program for healthy cooking and eating. With my simple-to-follow lists, he learned the principles of weight loss nutrition that he would not have explored or learned on his own. "I do not feel restricted but rather feel that I have been opened up to a whole new world of food," he told me. Andy went from 165 pounds to 135 pounds in 13 weeks. His energy improved, and his joint pain eased.

He was one of my clients who understood the core message from this program—fresh air living. The following simple statement helped him to make the right food decisions before ordering or going shopping: Eat as close as possible to the earth. By doing this, he realized how food advertising and his family influenced his choices. He also learned the role sugar played in his life. Today he enjoys preparing his own foods, eating foods that are on the list when eating out, and the abundance of energy he has because of a healthier, youn-ger, and stronger body. After going through the green-cleaning process from the outside to the inside and ridding himself from toxins and speeding up his digestion with Alpine foods, the compliments started. "What are you doing?" "Who is your doctor?" His skin improved from the inside out. His pains eased because of anti-inflammatory components in the Alpine foods. Overall he looked, felt, and moved like a 20-year-old.

Forbidden Fruit?

You may have noticed that fruits did not appear in any of the lists above. The reason is that they are higher in sugar and staying away from them for the first two weeks of better-choice eating can help you maintain the healthy blood sugar levels important in a weight loss program. But there is more to it. Many of us have been overindulging in simple processed sugars and simple natural

FAT LOSS: GRAINS VS. GREENS

Let us compare grains and vegetables. Despite all you read about "healthy" or "high-fiber" grains, they are not nearly as healthy or nutritionally complete as vegetables. In fact, grains are higher on the glycemic index than any common vegetable. That means they raise blood sugar levels, which should be kept steady when your goal is to lose fat, drop weight, or stay in a weight maintenance program.

Let us compare and contrast just a few grains and greens. These numbers were taken from the Glycemic Food Chart database (www.glycemicindex.com).

Grains: Whole-grain bread low 50 Rice, brown medium 55
All Bran low 42
Vegetables: Asparagus low 15 Lettuce low 15
Peppers low 15

As you can see, even if grains fall into the low category in the glycemic index, they still have higher numbers than vegetables. But there is more to consider. Vegetables provide—without a doubt— more vitamins, minerals, enzymes, and fiber per serving than grains. More fiber helps you regulate your blood sugar levels and prevent cardiovascular disease and cancer. Enzymes maintain all of our body functions. (Note to self: Eat veggies raw whenever possible.) Their vital enzymes are deactivated in heat above 118°F. Vitamins and minerals are vital for our immune system to function efficiently. You just get more bang for the buck with vegetables. And greens are less calorie dense than grains. That means you can eat more of them to feel fuller without gaining weight. If you eat the same amount of grains, you take in more calories and gain weight. Sorry.

Historically, the natural diet of humans was food that was picked, gathered, caught, or hunted. But as civilization evolved, cultivation of crops, or agriculture, was invented. And agriculture allowed us to flourish. Without those crops, the planet would not be able to support six billion people.

So are all grains bad? *No, but if your goal is weight loss, I recommend that you choose a carbohydrate that is fibrous (vegetables) over starchy (grains and some root vegetables). And do you want to wipe out grains off the earth? No, but it's important to choose grains wisely in your weight loss program and be aware of how many you eat in a day.*

sugars that yeast loves to feast on. Yeast is a fungus, and an overgrowth of yeast in your system is known as candida or yeast infections. Candida and other fungi produce a large number of biologically active substances called mycotoxins. These toxins are secreted to protect may fungi against viruses, bacteria, parasites, insects, animals, and humans. In our system, these mycotoxins can get into the bloodstream and produce an array of central nervous system symptoms such as fatigue, spaciness, confusion, irritability, mental fogginess, memory loss, depression, dizziness, mood swings, headaches, nausea—many of the signs and symptoms that are similar to low blood sugar.

Evidence now exists that fungi may initiate many degenerative diseases such as cancer, heart disease, gout, arthritis, and autoimmune disease such as chronic fatigue syndrome, multiple sclerosis, lupus, and rheumatoid arthritis. Many killer diseases are intimately connected to fungal connection. Hence our job is to prevent this and cleanse our bodies of fungal infection to rid us of mycotoxins.

Additionally, many foods that have been considered typically helpful have been discovered to be heavily colonized by fungi and their mycotoxins. That is why you will find corn, peanuts, cashews, and dried coconut in the Stay Away From category. Processed sugar as well as simple sugars from fruits feeds the fungi. You want to experience a clean system. You will know it when you feel a resurgence of energy and optimism. After 14 days, you can add fruit into the rotation, as listed below.

At first, eat only from the Best and Good fruit categories for 7 days. Then add category Stay Away From fruits. This strategy is important as well in the *A Flat Belly – "Schnell" (fast)!* program that you will read in chapter 8 (page 119).

FRUITS

The Most Beneficial	Beneficial	Stay Away From
Lemons (juice)	Avocados	Blackberries
Limes (juice)	(one a week)	Blueberries
	Cranberries	Boysenberries
	(raw or cooked)	Raspberries
	White Grapefruits	Apples
		Apricots
		Bananas
		Canned Fruits
		Cantaloupe Melons
		Cherries
		Currants
		Dates
		Dried Fruits (any kind)
		Figs
		Fruit Juice (except those in Category 1 and 2)
		Grapes
		Guavas
		Kiwis
		Mangoes
		Nectarines
		Oranges & Tangerines
		Olives
		Papayas
		Peaches
		Pears
		Pineapples
		Pink or Red Grapefruits
		Plums
		Pomegranates
		Prunes & Raisins
		Watermelon

1
2
3
4
5
6
7
8
9
10
11

How to Take the Next Bite

This is an eating plan you can use for years because it will help you maintain your weight and healthy eating. Some people stay on the Fresh Air Foods weight-loss eating program for life, making minor adjustments to suit their tastes. Others opt to come back to this phase periodically, when they have put on a little weight, see dark circles under the eyes, or simply need to get refocused on their health and appearance. For best results, as mentioned, avoid fruit for 14 days. After that, add fruits gradually as a treat. For easy to prepare and delicious recipes that follow the categories, go to chapter 10, *Hudry Wusch: Eat Yourself Thin*.

Jump-Start Your Weight Loss

Some of us need more structure to see instant results. If you crave structure, here is a 3-day sample plan that you can easily follow. In this phase, you can eat 1,300 to 1,500 calories providing you are active 3 to 5 days a week. If you are less active, eat slightly less.

If you are in a maintenance phase, after achieving your goal or the 14 days, you can reintroduce quality red meat 2 or 3 times a month. This is especially important for women as they lose iron during their menstrual cycle.

We are individuals and each of us has a different genetic makeup and goals. After years of experience, I discovered the best ratios among carbohydrates, protein, and fat for weight loss. This ratio is a 40-40-20 ratio. The sample menus below are written with a 40-40-20-nutrition ratio. Some will do better than others with this ratio. The key is to change the ratios while tracking and measuring your success to see if they are working for you. You can change from 40-40-20 to 50-30-20, 40-30-30, or to 30-40-30. This will give you the best feedback regarding what works best for your body type.

Sample Menus for Alpine Eating with Fresh Air Foods

DAY ONE

Alpine Eye-Opener:
1 glass water with fresh lemon
Peppermint tea

Breakfast
½ cup oatmeal made with brown rice milk and cinnamon
8 oz nonf. yogurt with 1 cup blueberries
6 almonds

Snack 1
8 oz nonf. yogurt

Lunch
Salad with:
½ cup onions
1 beet
1 ½ cups cooked squash, summer
2 cups broccoli
4 cups lettuce
3 sardines
¼ cup quinoa
2 tsp olive oil and lemon juice

Snack 2
2 hard-boiled eggs or egg salad

Dinner
20 med. spears asparagus
4 oz organic grilled chicken with lemon
½ avocado

DAY TWO

Alpine Eye-Opener:
1 glass water with fresh lemon
Peppermint tea

Breakfast
8 oz nonf. yogurt
1 cup blueberries
12 almonds
1 oz flaxseed, ground

Snack 1
½ grapefruit

Lunch
Salad with:
½ cup sprouts
2 cups lettuce
1 cup tomatoes
1 cup peppers
1 cup kale
4 cups spinach
¼ cup millet
1 tsp oil and lemon juice

Snack 2
1 whole egg

Dinner
6 oz chicken breast
1 cup kohlrabi
½ avocado
½ grapefruit

DAY THREE

Alpine Eye-Opener:
1 glass water with fresh lemon
Peppermint tea

Breakfast
½ cup oatmeal
8 oz nonf. yogurt
1 tsp raw almond butter
1 oz flaxseed, ground

Snack 1
1 cup fresh cut kohlrabi

Lunch
2 cups kale
½ cup onion
1 cup beets
1 cup celery
1 large artichoke
1 bunch spinach
¼ cup quinoa
1 tsp olive oil and lemon juice

Snack 2
Egg salad with rye bread

Dinner
4 oz wild salmon
2 cup zucchini
½ avocado

1
2
3
4
5
6
7
8
9
10
11

Worksheet 6

Still not sure? Good things take training and so does your decision-making process. Start with smaller steps. When you eat out, pick turkey burgers over beef burgers. Choose cheese from grass-fed animals over cheese from conventionally raised animals. Pick fruit sorbet over chocolate ice cream and freshly squeezed fruit juice over soda. Pick whole wheat pasta over white pasta. These changes are small but big in the overall results. Write down the foods that you eat on a regular basis that are in the Stay Away From category; next to it, write the better option that you will choose.

Stay Away From Foods   **Your Better Option**

1. ....

2. ....

3. ....

4. ....

5. ....

6. ....

7. ....

Get ready. It is going to be a lovely (and delicious!) ride. You will experience the positive effects of this type of eating almost immediately. Any bloating or heaviness in your stomach will disappear, so you will soon be sporting a flat belly. The dark circles under the eyes will slowly disappear. Friends, colleagues, family, and even strangers will remark on the glow of your skin. With time, your most recalcitrant fat—in your waist and in your butt—will finally start melting away. But most importantly, you will start to love yourself again when looking into your own eyes in the mirror.

ALPINE
WEIGHT LOSS
SECRETS

8 Ways to Start Today

You might be saying, "Sounds good. Maybe I will try it tomorrow." Do not put this off. Do not tell yourself some day. Some day is today. Stop, pause, and breathe. Now make the decision that you will start today. Write it in your calendar. It can be so empowering to see a string of days where you have noted "I did not eat chips" or "Had a salad today." Here is how easy it can be to start the change happening in your life today.

❶   **Order tomatoes instead of potatoes.** The next time you are ordering breakfast, tell the waiter you want tomatoes instead of the fried potatoes. It is an easy move that can save you lots of calories.

❷   **3-day success and 1-day reward.** Move it forward with an approach to stick to the program for just 3 days. Use the fourth day to reward yourself with what you like. And then come back to it. Moving it forward this way takes off the pressure and lets you celebrate success. Gradually increase the 3 days to longer intervals or reward yourself only once on the fourth day.

❸   **Cooking pasta?** In the last minutes of cooking time, stir in ribbons of summer squash or zucchini with your pasta. The result: less pasta and more vegetables!

❹   **Explore and discover.** Just add one new food item per week. Taste something that you thought you would hate but really don't know. Go out of your comfort zone. Try a new vegetable. Find a way that you can work with it.

❺   **Eat better fat.** Burn fat by eating fat. Not just any kind of fat. Brown adipose tissue burns white fat tissue. Studies have shown that by increasing intake of unsaturated fats such as olive oil, flaxseed, black currant seed oil, and pumpkin seed oil, brown tissue is stimulated and burns up to 10% more fat.

❻   **Go green, go grass fed.** When you eat grass-fed meat, you will be getting lots of conjugated linoleic acid, which stimulates weight loss. It has also been shown that by consuming grass-fed protein versus conventional protein, weight loss is easier to maintain. Conventionally raised livestock is fed grain, which decreases linoleic acid content by up to 80%.

❼   **Have butter, not margarine!** Pass up the margarine or butter-like spreads in favor of the real thing. Researchers from the University of Wisconsin believe that we are missing a vital source of conjugated linoleic acid (a natural fat-burner and weight loss chemical) because we are told to avoid full-fat dairy products like butter and yogurt.

8   **Work with your habit.** Say you have a habit of going in the fridge to look for food. Instead of trying to stop it altogether (that is really tough), simply turn it into a good-for-you thing. Fill bottles with water and flavor them with fruits, ginger, lemon, or tea. Reach for them and drink them instead of soda. The coldness will be refreshing and stimulating, helping you to refocus on your work.

Chapter 4

IMPROVE YOUR FAT-TITUDE

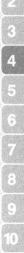

Why Certain Foods Can Make You Fat

Back home, we have a saying that's often used when making a New Year's resolution: *Weg mit dem Speck*. Loosely translated this would be "Lose the bacon" or "Out with the fat!" It makes sense. Too much of anything can result in weight gain. Now's the time to trim the excess "bacon" from your diet, your activity decisions, and your life. First, let's consider diet.

You know these bad boys: alcohol, white sugar, white flour, white rice, caffeine, and yeast. From my point of view, these are threats to your success. These damaging, empty calories will work against you because these foods actually require more nutrients to be digested than they provide, depleting your body rather than nourishing it. These foods put you on a fast track to aging, weight gain, and a slower metabolism.

Alcohol

Alcohol causes inflammation of your digestive organs, bloating, and fatigue. It's a diuretic and takes more enzymes and vitamins to process than it contributes to your body. Drinking too much also taxes the liver and increases abdominal fat since alcohol readily converts to fat. Yes, new research has shown that red wine contains high amounts of antioxidants and the phytochemical resveratrol, an anti-inflammatory. But there's also a downside. Alcohol also lowers your inhibition, which can undermine your decision-making process and lead to less-than-ideal choices. Once you complete the 14-day Alpine Eating Plan, reintroduce 1 glass or 2 a week if you must. When you do so, pay attention how you feel. If it makes you bloated, you might want to stay away from alcohol and save it for special occasions.

Also remember that 1 glass of wine has about 120 calories. Just 1 glass of wine each night adds up to 840 calories in a week and 3,360 calories in a month. 3,500 calories makes about 1 pound. In 1 year, if you maintain the nutrition required by your BMR (basal metabolic rate) and add on only 1 drink per day, you can gain 12 pounds per year. Keep in mind that your metabolism slows down every decade by 2% after the age of 25. An easy Alpine solution to this is to have a spritzer. Back home we use half of a glass of white wine and half of a glass of mineral water. The alcohol and the calories are diluted by 50%. This simple strategy can help you lose 50% of the anticipated weight gain.

BREAK THAT SUGAR HABIT

Here's a simple strategy. Replace white sugar, brown sugar, evaporated cane juice, corn syrup, and so on with natural fruit sugars. Your best to worse choices are:

* Fruit
* Food sweetened with fruit juice
* Amazake, malted grains, brown rice syrup, or agave syrup
* Molasses
* Honey or maple syrup
* Fructose

Refined Carbohydrates – Simple Sugars

The most commonly consumed simple sugars are whites: flour, sugar, and rice. Their lack of fiber has a detrimental effect on insulin levels. If that weren't bad enough, these foods do not provide sufficient nutrients to create the chemical reactions triggered by trace minerals and vitamins that lead to health and a younger-looking you. Instead, eating them leads to fatigue, dizziness, low energy, and weight gain.

Eating these calories leaves you wanting more because your cells are not nourished, which means you don't achieve the healthy feeling of satisfaction that you get by eating the more wholesome versions such as brown rice, whole grain pasta, and sugars from unaltered natural sources such as fruits and raw honey.

Caffeine

Caffeine causes "adrenal fatigue," in which your adrenal glands over-produce the hormone cortisol, which controls how your body metabolizes fat, protein, and carbohydrates. High cortisol levels slow down cell healing and regeneration and impair vital hormones that aid in digestion, metabolism, and mental function. Caffeine also interferes with healthy endocrine function and weakens your immune system. This is just the start; there is more to it.

In 2007, more information began to appear on food labels. Caffeine was added. Now we can see how much caffeine we are getting, and many of us don't know anything about the good, the bad, and the ugly when it comes to caffeine. Here is the quick breakdown.

The Good: A Quick Pick-Me-Up – First, caffeine is not just found in coffee; it can be found in sodas and chocolate. Also, don't forget it can be found in those energy drinks and some over-the-counter medicines. The problem is not that you consume caffeine but rather the amount you consume and your reaction to it.

The good thing about caffeine is that it is a central nervous system stimulant. It increases your basal metabolic rate, which helps you burn more calories (although exercise is still the most effective as it helps in stress management, building up lean muscle tissue to stay strong, and to burn more calories). It temporarily increases your mental clarity, as well as your muscular coordination for activities like typing. If you are one of many individuals dealing with breathing problems, you should probably also know that caffeine can open up air passages and helps increase respiration rates. If you have low blood pressure, caffeine can also be a simple way to give it a modest boost. Overall, a dosage of 50 to 100 mg of caffeine can have a stimulating effect on your system and increase your daily functions.

The Bad: An Addictive Fix – However, not all of the news is good. If taken in excess, caffeine can be addictive; to receive the same jolt you get when you first start taking it, you need to gradually increase your dose. Studies have shown that tiredness introduced by caffeine withdrawal can be fixed by additional caffeine intake.

So you should ask yourself: When I am tired and reaching for my caffeine fix, am I giving myself energy or am I managing the withdrawal effect? Studies have shown that the so-called pick-me-up effect is often actually a managing of withdrawal effects springing from addiction to caffeine.

The Ugly: A Body Out of Balance – When caffeine is used in excess, your body's own mechanisms do not work as they are intended to. Your hormone levels go out of whack, leading to such symptoms as excess nervousness, irritability, insomnia, dizziness, extreme fatigue, headaches, heartburn, anxiety, hypertension, and palpitations. It's enough, frankly, to make you dizzy. But this is not the whole story.

One of the other issues is the presence of tannic acid, a mild gastrointestinal irritant, in many caffeinated beverages. Get too much of this, and it will hinder the proper absorption of nutrients and minerals that your body needs for proper functioning. These losses most likely will not be replaced with normal nutritional intake.

Many caffeinated beverages also come part and parcel with another stimulant—sugar. For some, excessive sugar intake can over-stimulate the adrenal glands, and persistent usage can even weaken them. When your adrenal glands do not function well, fatigue sets in. Sugar and caffeine will do little to help to increase your energy.

How Much Is Too Much? – A high intake of caffeine is 500 mg daily. A medium intake is between 250 and 500 mg and a low intake is below 250 mg. The following list of beverages and foods, along with the amount of caffeine in each serving, will help you determine the category you fall into:

Coca Cola Classic	34.5 mg (12-ounce can)
Diet Pepsi	36 mg (12-ounce can)
Pepsi	37.5 mg (12-ounce can)
Diet Coke	46.5 mg (12-ounce can)
Mountain Dew	54 mg (12-ounce can)
Diet Pepsi Max	69 mg (12-ounce can)
Instant Coffee	40-105 mg (150 ml cup)
Filtered Coffee	110-150 mg (150 ml cup)
Tea	20-100 mg (150 ml cup)
Starbucks Coffee, Grande	500 mg (16-ounce cup)
Chocolate Cake	20-30 mg (one slice)
Caffeine Pill	50-200 mg (read label to determine exact dose)

Add up your daily intake of these beverages to determine how much caffeine you're getting.

Even if your total is below 500 mg, it may not be time to breathe a sigh of relief just yet. The negative effects mentioned above can occur with as little as 100 mg of caffeine intake daily. We are individuals, and everyone reacts differently. So if you think you might have issues with excessive caffeine consumption, you might want to taper your intake for 14 days and let your adrenal glands recover to have a fully functioning metabolism. The best solution is to commit yourself to a lifestyle that focuses on exercise and proper nutritional intake to perform, stay energized, and to look your best.

Yeast

I'm sure you've heard about yeast infections. Yeast and other fungi produce a large number of toxins. When they get into your bloodstream, fatigue, memory loss, dizziness, headaches, and mental fogginess can occur. What feeds the yeast in your body is the yeast in bread, along with foods that are stored or fermented. Sugar also feeds yeast.

Taming Withdrawal Symptoms: Dealing with Sugar Shock, Caffeine Cutoffs, and Alcohol Avoidance

If you've been eating mostly refined sugars and drinking caffeine and alcohol for years, your adrenal glands may be over-stimulated and not functioning efficiently. Also, whenever you consume too much sugar, your insulin levels surge, which puts your system in overdrive and leaves you constantly craving more food to boost your energy levels. Even a good night's sleep may not give you the rest and rejuvenation that you're looking for.

During the initial stages, your body may experience withdrawal symptoms, including headaches, fatigue, slight shakiness, mild tremors, disorientation, diarrhea, sweating, hot and cold flashes, fatigue, and decreased mental performance. Don't worry. Your body is just cleaning itself out so that it can run better in the future.

To combat any symptoms you experience, I highly recommend doing moderate exercise such as walking, biking, or swimming. Getting a lot of sleep also helps. Ideally, go to bed at 10:30 P.M. and get up between 5:30 and 6:00 A.M. Sneak in a 10-minute nap. You might want to take some vitamin C, B 100 complex, and a good multivitamin. The bottom line: listen to your body. Your energy will return shortly and you'll feel much stronger.

One Thing You CAN Eat: More Fat!

It sounds counterintuitive, but to burn fat, you have to eat fat. Specifically, fat that is high in gamma linolenic acid burns a specific form of body fat known as brown fat. This fat type surrounds your vital organs such as the kidneys, heart, and adrenal glands. It also cushions your spinal column, neck, and major thoracic blood vessels. Gamma linolenic acid is a precursor of prostaglandins, which regulate the brown adipose tissue by acting as a catalyst to either turn it on or off, incinerating other types of fat in the body.

In Europe, we are used to consuming evening primrose oil for many health-related issues. Similarly, we use flaxseed oil often—it is another one that is high in gamma linolenic acids and high in omega 3 and omega 6 fatty acids. The best fat-loss results have been accomplished with adding one teaspoon of evening primrose oil or two teaspoons of ground flaxseeds to your morning breakfast.

Lose Your Mental Fat Too!

Let's get rid of your mental fat. Yes, get rid of your lazy, I don't want to do it, or I am too tired and don't have time mental fat. It's holding you back from accomplishing your goals. Get up and replace your clogging mental fat with fluid oil. Let it run. Make it move. Don't get mentally lazy and clog yourself with mental fat.

A good place to start: listen to your own excuses. Some of the best I've heard that you might be using as well:

- "I am healthy. I don't need to exercise."
  Diseases don't occur overnight. Only the diagnosis does.

- "I still fit into my jeans from 5 years ago."
  Yes, but how about 20 years ago?

- "My cholesterol is low. I am fine."
  This is not the only measurement of health.

- "My doctor said I am healthy."
  Did he measure your muscular and cardio strength?

- "I have a pain in my hip."
  Sure that is a reason, but it leaves you with your upper body and midbody still able to exercise. Just bring it down to your level, so that you work in a painfree environment.

The biggest mental fat is not to work to overcome your challenges. The challenge in an exercise program is to find what keeps it interesting for you and what makes it exciting, so that it is not just another task. Make it fun and concentrate on a feeling of accomplishment. Just go in a gym and see failure in people's faces. People look bored on the treadmill, on the bike, or with their trainer. Like robots. Come on, what a shame. Take a challenge once a week to take your workout to the next level. Push yourself; you just might fire yourself up.

Worksheet 7

What is too much in your life right now? This is different for everyone as all of us have different circumstances. To give you some ideas, here are some suggestions: Might it be food? Inactivity? Perhaps too much eating out? Going out? Fill out below what your current mental fats are. Then come up with a strategy next to it for getting rid of excessive mental fat that slows you down.

Current mental fat:

....

....

....

....

....

....

Strategy to lose your mental fat:

....

....

....

....

....

....

This is just one part of it. There might also be stress, boredom, and no excitement in your life. That is all mental fat that slows you down. Ask yourself what kind of stress affects you so you eat off the chart. Might it be physical, emotional, work, or family related? Identify the sources of stress that upset you and make you comfort yourself with food. Write down the kind of stress that affects you and below that a solution to neutralize it.

ALPINE
WEIGHT LOSS
SECRETS

Stress factor number 1:

....

....

....

....

Prevention:

....

....

....

....

....

....

Stress factor number 2:

....

....

....

....

Prevention:

....

....

....

....

....

ALPINE
WEIGHT LOSS
SECRETS

Stress factor number 3:

....

....

....

....

Prevention:

....

....

....

....

....

Stress factor number 4:

....

....

....

....

Prevention:

....

....

....

....

....

Stress factor number 5:

....

....

....

....

Prevention:

....

....

....

....

....

Boredom with your life can be another type of mental fat. For example, not being happy with your accomplishments. Food is the only joy that gives you excitement, and you look forward to eating. Think hard. Is there another spark that you can light that makes you jump out of bed in the morning to get it done again? Write down below what currently bores you. Then write below what you can do to change this.

What bores you?

....

....

....

....

What can you do to change this?

....

....

ALPINE
WEIGHT LOSS
SECRETS

Listen to yourself. What excuses do you come up with to not do what is asked here? Are you turning questions in such a way that you just don't have to answer them? Come, be honest with yourself. You can do this for yourself. This is one of the worst mental fats you can encounter, and this is the hardest to get rid of. Why? Because it can be a pattern, a personality pattern, that needs to be changed. And this is simple. Capitalize by changing your communication from I can't to I can.

My excuse number 1:

....

....

....

....

Replacement:

....

....

....

....

My excuse number 2:

....

....

....

....

Replacement:

....

....

....

My excuse number 3:

....

....

....

....

Replacement:

....

....

....

....

My excuse number 4:

....

....

....

....

Replacement:

....

....

....

....

ALPINE
WEIGHT LOSS
SECRETS

My excuse number 5:

....

....

....

....

Replacement:

....

....

....

....

Mental fat is sticky. It slows you down. It doesn't move you forward or in the right direction. Get rid of this fat. And sometimes, you need a kick in the backside to do exactly that.

1
2
3
4
5
6
7
8
9
10
11

Blew it? 10 Ways to Get Back on Track

❶ **Read the label.** No, you should not be interested in the percentage of fat, how much sugar, and how many vitamins are in that product. Instead, pay attention to the ingredients list. For example, you will find labels that have 0 fat calories. But to make it taste good, chemicals and sugars are added as main ingredients in that product. The amount of ingredients is listed in descending order. A simple rule: If you can say it, don't eat it.

❷ **Fill it full and don't leave it half empty.** Okay, you like alcohol. I understand. Add on instead of remove. We in Europe enjoy a spritzer, which is half white wine and half sparkling water. Refreshing in the summer and fewer calories.

❸ **Explore and discover.** Used to cereals in the morning? White pasta for lunch? White rice for dinner? Try replacements. The brand Ezekiel 4:9 makes fantastic breakfast cereals without the refined carbohydrates and sugars. Try whole wheat, brown rice, spelt, or quinoa pasta instead of white pasta. There are so many options available. Find one you like. What to do in a restaurant? Remember, "Pick tomatoes and not potatoes." Practice your decision-making skills.

❹ **Drink up.** Morning is a time to wake up and enjoy a routine that you might have. And routines are habits. So you might be back on 5 cups of coffee per day. Do the following. Try decaf coffee over regular coffee—just 1 a day. Try black tea over coffee and peppermint tea over black tea. Keep the routine. Keep it hot. And let your body wake up instead of fire up the minute you wake up.

❺ **White out and color in.** Look at your plate as an artist's palette. There are white breads or brown breads, black coffee or brown coffee, butter or better butter. Frankly, it sounds a little dull and monotonous, right? So change it. Choose green, red, and orange. Or blue, yellow, and light green. Have 3 colors with each meal instead of just white, brown, or black. Keep it simple by just adding green for lunch and dinner. Then add blue and yellow for breakfast. And so on. Raw would be best over fried or boiled.

❻ **Interrupt your stress pattern.** Stress is a killer to your diet. Manage your stress. Instead of food, reach for your sneakers. Don't think. Put them on and go for a walk, run, or to the gym. Continue the second and third day until it becomes your routine.

❼ **Ditch the disturbia.** By this I mean anything that brings you into a disturbing state. It might be an argument. Take the first step. Say that you are sorry. What do you have to lose besides additional pounds? Maybe it's the internal argument you have, trying not to stop by the candy store on the way home. Change your route to avoid temptation. Or accept that you screwed up. Acceptance brings the power of control. Get right back to your statement "Why I want to accomplish this goal."

❽ **Reevaluate your emotions.** You let it go. Your emotions control you again. Whip out your diary and write down what is going on. If you can track progress, you can measure it. If you can measure it, you can control it.

❾ **Schedule your *Flat Belly – "Schnell" (fast)!* day.** This is a very short-term approach that I have taught many clients with great success. Take your calendar and schedule your day. Stick to it. This quick jump-start may be just what you need.

❿ **Sweat today.** Don't schedule a day in the future when you'll start exercising. Do it now. A motion creates momentum. You don't need to hire the best trainer or join a gym. Start the momentum right in your home.

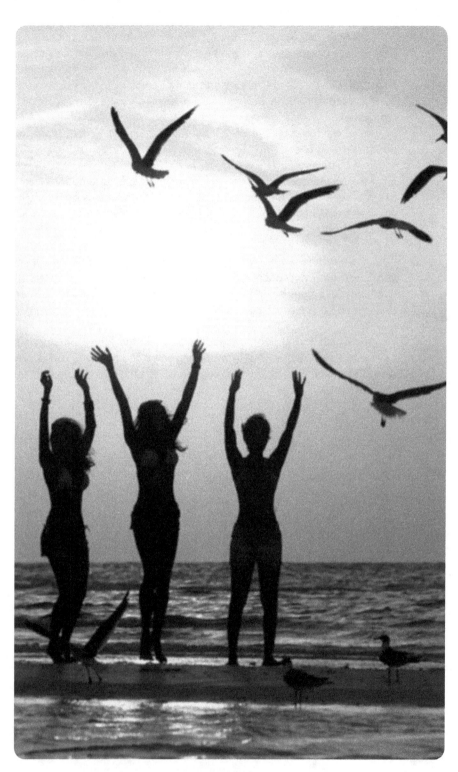

ALPINE
WEIGHT LOSS
SECRETS

Chapter 5

INSTANT ANTI-AGER: YOUR POSTURE

1
2
3
4
5
6
7
8
9
10
11

Posture That Ages You

Times have changed. Our unnatural sedentary lifestyle, which has become second nature to tens of millions of us, is aging us prematurely. It shows in our fitness level, health, appearance, and aging process. Today, we have pain in our lower backs, shoulders, and hips. Quite frankly, I never heard about these issues as I grew up. Even older people were active in the forest, fields, or the mountains.

We are meant to be constantly active and out in the open air in nature as much as possible. We're not designed to sit for hours, which changes our bodies' natural alignment and throws the central nervous system out of kilter. But today most of our jobs require that we sit in offices in front of computers for hours at a time. That usually means you're sitting hunched over in front of your computer screen with a forward-headed body posture, an arched lower back, and without any contraction of the abdominal wall. That's an unnatural position for your spine and the muscle groups around the spinal cord. Your muscles and ligaments don't have the right tension (I'll explain this below), and they press on the nerves. This is also particularly true for women who wear high heels.

That's why so many people have injuries in the cervical spine and lumbar spine, and why you so often hear people complaining that "My neck hurts" or "My lower back hurts." Or why you may feel a pain in your hamstring or hip as you exercise or walk down the street. This kind of persistent discomfort can make you feel like you've aged 20 years. It also makes you skeptical that you can ever be really physically active again.

When you are fully coordinated and pain free, you can reclaim the joy of moving freely and being active even late into old age. I want you to run with wild abandon again, something you might have not done since you were a child. And is it not time to change your dress size from 12 to 6 and maybe even smaller? Correct your posture to make you look young and move pain free again!

Reboot Your Central Nervous System:

Alignment, Activation, and Elongation

An inactive person who has little strength in the legs, mid-body, or upper body needs to reprogram the faulty or badly learned functions of her body so that she can perform a proper lunge, squat, or mid-body exercises. And yes, even if you've been working out for years, you may be using incorrect technique or form that's resulted in pain and damaging wear and tear in your joints and muscles and also in your organs. In either case your central nervous system needs reprogramming.

The central nervous system is comprised of your brain and spinal cord, and it controls and coordinates all your movements. Each of us learns a certain way to walk, talk, and think from childhood, so we run like a computer with certain software. If you have not learned how to contract your abdominal wall, for instance, you need to get that software and start running it on your computer, otherwise known as your brain. After doing the movement over and over again, it will become second nature, and you'll increase your performance capability and strength. But first, you need help building your new software, which the Alignment, Activation, and Elongation (AAEs) will help you do.

There might be many reasons why some people might have a faulty posture. The AAEs are a great start to correct slight deviations from a correct posture. Yet the AAEs are not designed for individuals who are dealing with more severe cases of misalignments. It is best to work with a qualified professional who can assess and give you corrective exercises, some of which you will learn about here.

It takes 365 repetitions to recondition your central nervous system, but it only takes 10 to 15 repetitions to recondition it incorrectly again. So there's a learning curve. You have to do it over and over again the right way. Some people can't do 10 repetitions correctly. They can only do one or two. If the third is wrong, you've got to start over, so slow everything down and get it right. If you have to change position slightly, turn the knee out a little more to make the adjustment. Don't move forward on the other exercises in phase 2 until you've mastered the proper form. If you experience pain in your back or knees later on, you'll now know how to fix it.

Correct your alignment, activation, and elongation throughout the day while you're sitting, exercising, or walking down the street. You need to create new connections in your brain in order to execute movements correctly and without pain so that you can stay active as many Austrians do even into old age. This program is not something you do once and then move on to another chapter. The pages of this chapter should be dog-eared!

Instant Age Loss: Back to Balance

When we speak about posture, we need to address the balance of the muscular system. This is a simple concept that you will need to understand to improve and correct your posture. Your body functions much like a bicycle wheel. Picture a bicycle wheel that has a frame and spokes attached to it.

When the same amount of tension is applied to the spokes of the bicycle wheel, it runs very smoothly.

However, what happens when one spoke is tighter than another, and thus stronger? The bicycle wheel starts to wobble. It doesn't function properly.

Looks like the number 8 from the front—it's out of alignment.

That's what happens when some of your muscles are weaker and others are stronger. Your body is out of alignment, without the drive and the power to execute movement properly. You feel weak and very slow, so it's important to correct muscular imbalances and improve your range of motion. If you have a wider range of motion, you're able to achieve a larger muscular contraction. In other words, you're building up more lean muscular tissue, which means you're burning more calories. The result? Bigger weight loss. Isn't this one of your objectives?

Flexibility keeps you young and agile. It gives your entire body more stability so you have freedom of movement. To improve balance in your muscular system, hold the stretches that feel tight on your muscles. When holding a stretch that doesn't feel tight to you, move on to the next. How to improve your flexibility?

**Go to www.AlpineWeightLossSecrets.com/BookBonusLogIn.html
and access your free bonus program.**

Alignment: Correct Posture for Pain-Free Results

We all want to be as strong as possible and able to execute movements from a position of strength. The key is alignment—putting the correct tension on the skeletal system so that it functions at 100% and allows you to perform movements as they are supposed to be executed.

I can guarantee that most individuals have skeletal issues because of muscle tension created by poor alignment. The spine consists of 24 bones, called vertebrae. Ligaments and muscles connect these bones together to form the spinal column. Without the spinal column, you couldn't stand up or keep yourself upright. It gives you the flexibility to bend and twist and reach. It also protects the spinal cord, a column of nerves that allows your brain to direct all the other parts of your body. The AAEs help create the alignment and activation necessary to stabilize the lumbar curve, which is the lower spine, the thoracic spine, the mid-back, and cervical spine, which starts just below your skull and is the critical juncture with the thoracic spine. When movements deviate from the natural alignment of the body, injuries can occur in the lower back, hips, knees, neck, and shoulders, which are the kinds of aches and pains that are often associated with old age.

Many people overlook alignment when working out or even just walking down the street. But whenever we move, our bodies must be correctly aligned in order to achieve the maximum benefit and prevent injuries. Take off your shoes, stand in front of a full-length mirror, and assess your current posture by checking:

- Your alignment from shoulder, to hip, to knee, to ankles, and to the toes from an anterior view.
- From your head, to your shoulder, to your lower back, hip, and knees, and your heels from a lateral view.
  Please note: *Extreme deviations from the mentioned alignment will need corrective exercises from a qualified personal trainer or specialist.*

STOP THINKING IN PARTS!

Everything is so specialized in medicine today, so doctors focus only on their areas of expertise because that's the way they've been trained. One doctor is in charge of your knees, another's taking care of your lower back, and you've got another for your neck.

Wouldn't it be useful to have all these specialists get together and analyze your body as a whole—your shoulder and neck alignment, how you move, the strength level in your core abdominals, legs and arms, etc? This way they could figure out exactly what's going on when you're experiencing pain in one specific area.

Perhaps the lack of abdominal activation is contributing to your lower back or your shoulder pain or neck pain. Or it might be the opposite. Is the shoulder pain contributing to your neck pain? Wouldn't it be worth looking at the entire body to diagnose a problem rather than just looking at specific parts?

Checkpoint: Alignment, Activation and Elongation

Checkpoint Alignment (front)

Sit down on the floor with your back and spine against the wall and straighten your legs.

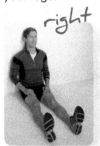
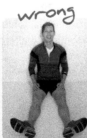

right   wrong

Flex your feet and align the toes, ankles, knees, hips, and shoulders in a straight line. Pay attention to how your feet are positioned. Are they turned out? Both or just one?
In either case, align your toes so that they are pointing straight up toward the ceiling—not inward or outward.

Adjust any deviation to this connective alignment as described above.

Keep this alignment when walking, running, sprinting, or performing exercises.

Checkpoint Alignment (side)

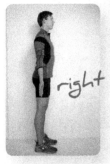

Stand straight and tall. Check whether your hip is aligned with your shoulder and your ankles when you look at your body from the side. To do this, simply push your hips forward while your back arches a little and your belly button comes out. Remember how this feels. It's the wrong way.

right

Push your hips back so that they are positioned directly over your heels. Can you feel that you have some activation in your abdominals? Not yet? Not a problem.

wrong

Keep the hip over your heels and just lean on your toes without lifting up your heels. Then shift your weight back on your heels again. One more time shift forward and pay attention to how your abdom-inals activate.

wrong

Notice that your hip is not shifting forward but rather your entire body, in alignment from your shoulder, hip, and heels, shifts forward. This is the activation that you want to maintain during exercise such as lunges, squats, runs, and sprints.

Checkpoint Activation: Strengthen Your Mid-body

Most people think of the mid-body as the abdominal muscles, but there's more to it. The mid-body consists of 6 main muscle regions, and each one has a particular function during movements such as lifting weights.

❶ The diaphragm separates the lungs from the digestive system and expands downward into the abdominal cavity during inhalation.

❷ The abdominal region includes your rectus abdominus, the internal and external obliques, your transverse abdominals, which is like an internal corset, and your inner and outer abdominal wall—all of which allows you to pull your stomach in and out.

❸ The pelvic girdle is the pelvic floor and the pelvic wall, which are at the bottom of your torso.

❹ Trunk extenders are the back muscles such as your quadratus lumborum (back extension), the multifidus, interspinales, and intertrans-versarii mediales, which act as an antagonist to the abdominals.

❺ Muscles of the chest and upper back are also considered the mid-body as they play an important role as well to stabilize the upper extremities. In the past, the muscles of the core were considered all the muscles as mentioned above, excluding the upper back and chest.

Generally, a sitting position creates an unstable environment because you're not activating your pelvic floor. You're relaxing! That pushes the stomach out. So when you stand up after a long period of sitting (year after year), you're not conditioned to maintain the activation of the abs and the pelvic floor. Then you start to move in an unstable position—your knee hurts, your hip hurts. It's all connected.

Checkpoint Activation: Pelvic Floor

Think of the pelvic girdle as your body's steering wheel. Pelvic girdle activation is often overlooked when it comes to exercise, but it provides critical stability for movement. When the muscles of the pelvic girdle are activated, you can control the movements of your hip and knees, which helps to create stability in the lower back, hips, and knees. It also tightens the muscles around the spine, which need to be stabilized in order to prevent injuries. Without the stability that mid-body strength provides, your back becomes a prime candidate for the sorts of injuries that are painful, costly, and make you feel about a hundred years old every time you move.

Practice 1

Think you need to go to the bathroom to pee. Really! Then, while peeing, simply stop and start again. Feel how your lower abdominal and pelvic girdle contracts when you stop. These are called Kegel exercises.

Practice holding this contraction while walking throughout the day. And, of course, during every minute of your exercise routine.

Checkpoint Activation: Abdominal Wall

Activation of the abdominal wall allows you to push the belly button out and pull it back in. If you push it out, you don't get the activation or tightening that creates stability for the spine.

The result? An unstable environment for movement. When you pull your belly button in, you're tightening all the muscles around your spine, which creates stability when you move. Otherwise you may get a herniated disk or other back issues.

Practice 2

Pull your belly toward your spine and try to hold this activation.

Practice both activations—the pelvic girdle and the abs—together.

However, keep in mind that they're inseparable. Both accommodate each other and work together.

Elongation: Think Tall

We've been talking a lot about creating stability around the spine but mostly from static positions such as when you're seated or standing straight against a wall. But how do you generate stability when you move? It's simple: make yourself a little taller. Try it now when you're sitting. Bring the shoulder blades down a bit. Do you feel the activation? If you make yourself longer, you're creating activation of all the little muscles around the spine that give you stability. Now you have a stabile environment for movement.

> ## PRACTICE YOUR KEGELS
>
> *Kegel exercises are not just squeezing your butt together or pulling your stomach in, and they're also not about pushing out and thrusting out your lower abdomen. Kegel exercises activate the pelvic girdle through an inward and up movement. This is not just for women! Guys, it's just as important for you, especially if you lift weights.*
>
> *You can find the deeper internal activations by using the muscles you use to stop the flow of urine. Be careful because you don't want to start actually retaining urine; it's just a way to help you identify the right muscles. You want to be able to hold the activation for 10 seconds, but you may have to work up to that. Try holding them six times a day.*
> *Do the Kegels anywhere, even while you're waiting on line at the supermarket. No one will ever know, but you'll be doing a world of good for your mid-body.*

Checkpoint: Elongation

Practice 3

Think tall. Simply imagine you have a string attached to the top of your head that pulls you up toward the sky.

Feel how your shoulders drop down.
Stay elongated throughout the day while sitting, walking, running, sprinting, or exercising.

Try to do all three activities at the same time while sitting: Align, Activate, and Elongate [AAEs]. Feel each single basic activation while sitting, as you did in the first position. Then practice AAEs while standing, walking, running, or lunging. Remind yourself throughout the day to focus on it.

ALPINE
WEIGHT LOSS
SECRETS

Worksheet 8

Posture is an important factor in how you are perceived by others. And the first impression always counts. Yes, you can improve your posture, but sometimes it is not your posture that needs adjustment. Sometimes it is your self-communication about life, how you think about yourself, your stage in life, and where you are going. Being upset, or perhaps depressed, can change your posture into forward-dropping shoulders, head down, eyes down, and a motionless facial expression.

Catch yourself and change it. If you think this might be you, go to chapter 9 and answer the 7 questions outlined there about *The Joy of Living: Think and Grow Thin!*

No matter what, practice your AAEs. Plan out specific times that you will implement them. For example, sitting in the office from 9:00 am to 9:03 am. Or walking from the office to the bus or car from 6:45 am to 6:55 am. The choice is yours.

Date	Time	Activity

AAE 1st: ....

AAE 2nd:..

AAE 3rd: ....

AAE 4th: ....

AAE 5th: ....

AAE 6th: ....

AAE 7th: ....

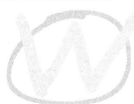

9 Anywhere, Anytime Posture Prompts

Correct posture is important to stay pain free, active, and look great at the same time. Check in with yourself and pay attention to what you do during the day with your body. Here are some check-ins to follow from morning till the evening to correct and improve your posture:

❶   **At the desk – Look at your workplace.** How is your computer positioned? Does it cause you to slump forward or tilt up your head to see the monitor? If yes, correct it so that your eyes are at the same level as the monitor. Raise the monitor with books, and if this is not possible, buy a chair that is adjustable to a lower or higher level.

❷   **Slumping – It is tiring to sit at a desk.** Pay attention to how you sit at a desk. Slumping? Feet up? Sure, it feels good, but if you do this every day for months, you will change your body's position, which will affect your posture and therefore your activity program. Remind yourself to sit upright, shoulders down, and head straight forward.

❸   **Telephone – I slept wrong and my neck hurts!** Or I hurt my neck and didn't know why! These are the lines that come up over and over again. Neck pain can have many sources. Yet check how you hold the telephone receiver. Perhaps between your head and your shoulder? Please buy a headset and start working with the headset. Even at home. This will free your hands to continue doing other work while you are speaking on the phone.

❹   **Get up – Sitting shortens your hamstrings.** And short hamstrings can change your pelvic position as the hamstring attaches in the ischial tuberosity (part of the pelvis). A short hamstring pulls your hip into a posterior tilt and causes a flat back. Get up and stretch your hamstrings. Remember, s/he who rests will rust.

❺   **The stretch – Slumping will lengthen your back musculature and shorten your chest and abdominals.** Remember the bicycle wheel analogy. What is short needs to get stretched, and what is long needs to get shortened. Stand up, weight on your heels, hands up toward the ceiling, flex your hands toward the back, and gently push the hips forward. A full-body stretch for your abs, chest, and hips while you are activating your glutes, back, and shoulders. Try to do this stretch at least twice a day.

ALPINE
WEIGHT LOSS
SECRETS

❻ **Your bags – Your bags can make or break your posture.**
More often than not, when a client consults me for a body analysis,
I find that one shoulder is higher than the other, creating neck
and shoulder problems. A simple strategy is to carry your bag on
both sides, switching it throughout the day or the journey. In fact,
carrying is a great way to practice your posture. Take 2 shopping
bags. Distribute the weight evenly and walk upright while pressing the
shoulders toward the heels. I call this the farmer's walk.

❼ **High heels – This is a big subject that can't be addressed in
detail here.** Here is the short version. High heels force your hips into an
anterior tilt, creating an increased lower back curvature. This is not all.
Because your body needs to adjust from a forward leaning posture into
an upright posture, you are forcing your head into a forward-headed
posture and rounded shoulders in extreme cases. The solution? Take
flat shoes with you when you go to work, walk short distances, and
address the issues that arise when wearing high heels.

❽ **Smile – Be happy.** Yes, be happy and change your body position. Snap out of feeling sorry of yourself and just walk tall. Be proud of
yourself. Pay attention to your own mental communication to yourself.
Negative communication on the inside will show up on the outside.

❾ **Walk proud – Accomplished something great?** Show it off
in your gestures. Your posture. I am sure you remember a time when
you were proud of yourself. Think back and remember how you walked
down the street. Just do it for fun. Practice being proud in your walk
and posture. Feel better instantly.

Before the start of an exercise program it's important to improve your posture.
Your posture is the core of the foundation needed for movement and increasing
resistance. Simple changes in your daily activity can and will make a difference.

1
2
3
4
5
6
7
8
9
10
11

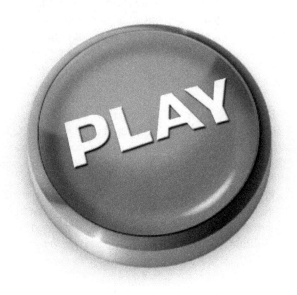

Chapter 6

THE AT-HOME ALPINE AEROBIC SOLUTION

Remember when you were a child and played for hours outdoors with your friends? You raced each other, competed, and plotted strategies to just have a good laugh. Your mind and body were totally engaged in whatever game or activity you were involved in. Your senses were, too. The fresh air, the sun, the wind, and perhaps rolling in the dirt were all part of the experience. When your mom called you to come in for lunch or dinner, you threw a fit. You wanted to keep going! Back home you felt happy, energized, and were looking forward to eating—and then heading back outdoors again.

Somewhere along the way, most people lose the simple delight in movement. Exercise becomes another dreaded task on the to-do list; joining a gym is punishment for an out-of-shape body. Did you know that treadmills originated in prisons as a way to get prisoners to exercise? No wonder so few of us look forward to going to the gym!

Push the Play Button

In my small village, there was always something physical to do. Most summer days we would ride our bikes over to our friend's house, which was a few villages and about five steep hills away, and then we'd race or go swimming. At harvest time, we helped farmers bring in their crops, hoisting bales of hay onto trucks, and crushing the grapes they grew. Most kids learned to ski and ice skate a day or two after they learned to walk, and so did I. (Okay, I'm exaggerating; it was really a week after!) It was just another way to stay active throughout winter. Looking back, I realize that my active, sports-filled childhood could not have been better training for the life I lead today as a fitness expert.

The older you get, the more difficult it will be to move. One of the reasons is that life just takes over. You give priority to your family, your work, making money, and just keeping your life going. Many times you forget to have fun. Then signing up to a gym might be the death curse to your resolve to stay active. You walk in and don't know what to do. So you just go from one station to the next. A personal trainer might help you to set up a program that focuses only on strength training but not movement conditioning. Many times this experience is boring. Are you surprised that individuals with a good New Year's resolution quit just after 4 weeks? The gym has its place. It is here for strengthening muscles against resistance heavier than your own body weight. This is a strategy to support your muscles, to stay strong and to be able to have fun with all the other activities that are to be discovered.

Find the fun in your activities again. It is always fun to improve as a group. You also can find classes that bring out the inner child when you participate in them. Do find the activity that you enjoy and not hate. Our current president plays basketball. Talk to him about basketball, and he will have an exciting conversation with you. He invites young college students to play with him. Then look at Oprah. She hates to run. She starts a gym program, and she stops. She doesn't have fun. She hates doing it on a continuous basis. The real solution for her would be to try different activities that she enjoys and doesn't hate to do. Do you find yourself in the same shoes? Then please stop what you do and find activities that you like to do and that bring you joy.

Here are some ideas for you:

Be silly at home. Who doesn't like to be silly? Make it fun. Get a dance DVD and follow it. Learn a dance step from a music video. What is even more fun is to look up the '80s music videos or tapes and do them from time to time.

Try out new activities. There is so much to discover. Trapeze, water polo, circus class, hand ball, dodgeball, basketball, volleyball, racketball, softball, tennis, golf, squash, and so many others. Go for the tryouts. Book yourself a beginner's lesson. Discover what is the most fun for you.

Fun with your friends. Get 5 friends together. Put each in charge of leading 1 exercise per day. If at a loss, there are so many ways to find workout ideas and programs on the Internet. Your benefit? Accountability! And unexpected workout activities that you might not have tried.

Join a hiking club. Hiking clubs meet regularly on the weekends or plan hiking trips to other areas. Best of all, many of them involve the entire family.

Join a running group. Benefit from the power of support. Women are fantastic supporters. They know how to help each other. And they know to say the right things to each other to keep going. Find a group that works for your needs. You might have to try out a few.

Suggest a parent and child class. Have you been in the situation where you dropped off your child and watched and waited for one hour until the activity was finished? Depending on the age of your child, you might suggest that an activity class could be created for mum/dad and children to stay active. Many times you can see that parents drop off their children for sports or play and just to sit and read or talk. This is a time you can use as well. And haven't you ever cracked up when children have fun with their toys? Fun, no? Join them.

The gym might be still your only place for activity. If this is your choice, then push the play button there. Don't sit around or wait for the machines. Use the toys that are available in the facility such as the jump ropes, the medicine balls, the ropes, the Swiss ball, and much more. Ask for help if you don't know how to use them. But start using the gym in such a way that brings variety and joy to your activity program.

Cynthia did it right. At one of the fitness promotion events for Adidas, she came to my table and asked how she could lose weight. We had a 5-minute conversation. During this time I took the time to encourage her to get started with friends or a group or make changes to her continuing program so that she keeps her muscles guessing what is coming next. She signed up for the free e-mini course "Look Better Slim," which is available on my Web site. She says it best in her own words:

"Dear Stefan,
I just wanted to let you know that I started working out on Jan 4, and I was around 187 lbs. Now I am down to 169, February 8. Thank you so much for all of your advice—I love it! Also, I go to the gym every day (almost—I rest on weekends or when I feel that my body needs it.) I always try to keep my body guessing. It's really fun, and I definitely watch what I eat because I value my body and health so much more since I have started working out. Thank you again for everything, your minicourse was motivational and inspiring!"

Cynthia

She managed to implement simple changes and have fun with a program that encourages her to push the play button. Having only spoken to her for 5 minutes, my curiosity wasn't satisfied. Why not just ask her exactly how she did it? And this was her answer, which is worth sharing with you:

"Hey Stefan,
Honestly, I just try different things. I never do the same routine more than three times a week; I change the incline and speed on the treadmill (interval), and I lift weights and do strength training. When I want some more fun I'll pop into a class or will go to the gym with a buddy. (Ex: my sister is coming with me tomorrow.) Most importantly, I try to keep it fun and always ask others for tips and advice. I keep an open mind because I think that I can learn from everyone. In terms of eating, I've included a lot more fish, I'm picky about which fats I want,

I dilute juices with water, I avoid soda and junk food, and I only eat a little white rice and pasta. I don't deprive myself, but I don't overeat either. I've also learned that a slice of cake never tastes as good as the first bite. So why eat the whole thing? This is what I have been doing so far, and I feel great, but I'm really scared that I will hit a plateau."

It took only a 5-minute conversation for her to change and to follow my simple instruction to have fun with whatever you do and start moving. And she does. The rest followed. She kept her program interesting to stick with it. Her next concern was that she reaches a plateau and her weight loss stops. This I will address in my Alpine Aerobics Solution program just below.

The Gym Without Walls

You don't have to go to the gym to get a good workout. Current scientific research recommends that you be active and exercise, but it doesn't tell you where to do it. Save your money. Learn a simple strategy that has been effective for decades back home. There, people maintain their athletic physiques without ever stepping foot in a gym. You too will discover what joy there is in simply moving your body on a daily basis.

The Alpine Aerobic Solution

My Alpine Aerobic Solution is designed to get you back to an active life-style. There's no gimmick. It's back to basics: you're using your own body weight instead of gym machines.

Most people who live in an Alpine environment do not think about aerobic activity. And I don't want you to think about it either. Rather, enjoy the environment around you while being active outside—the birds flying by, the blue sky and white clouds, the trees, the sun reflecting on the fields or water—and noticing new things along the way. These discoveries change from season to season—from new buds on a rose bush to the changing leaves in fall to meeting other people enjoying the same hiking trail. Time spent outdoors is full of surprises and unpredictability—a hill around the corner, a muddy puddle on a path, or a fallen tree. The connection to the present moment while being active is what brings you pleasure and joy.

You may need some attitude adjustment. A walk is not just a walk or an activity that burns calories. A walk is a moment to celebrate time for yourself when you're able to disconnect from all your obligations, worries, and pressures. Walking or hiking a mountain is a way to check in with yourself. Are you still in touch with your senses and life goals? Or are you so disconnected that you're not paying attention to your needs and real feelings? In some ways, walking and hiking are like an Alpine therapy session—for free! The environment listens and communicates with us while we're moving through it to enjoy new experiences. That's something a gym can't provide.

Aim to do the Alpine Aerobic Solution 1 to 2 times a week. Make it a pleasure, not a penance. Take time for yourself; enjoy being outside; discover new areas, neighborhoods, or trails; and celebrate yourself and nature. Everything is interconnected. Practice awareness when exploring the outdoors. The trees give us oxygen, the sun gives us heat and energy, and movement provides stress release. Bring your consciousness back to your environment, your life, and yourself.

Making the Most Of Your Alpine Aerobic Solution

The Alpine Aerobic Solution is a great strategy to stay active without a gym and it allows you to focus on your goals and yourself. And there is more to it.

Have you noticed, if you had the chance to visit Alpine environments, that many women there are size 0, 2, or 4? A conversation in a New York City elevator drove this point home. As I eavesdropped (yes, I did), I learned that this woman just returned from a trip. Stunned, she explained, "I just came back from Colorado, and can you believe that with my size 6, I was the fattest woman on the mountain? Everybody else was a size 0 or a size 2." There can be many reasons for this. Diet is one of them. The Alpine Eating Plan will help you to take this under control. Activity is another issue. Not just the activity alone—the intensity levels will impact the outcome as well. Individuals who live in Alpine environments do have the Alpine Advantage, which is the natural environment of uphill and downhill walking or hiking. This change of elevation to walk, hike, or run is fun, challenging, and burns not just the highest number of calories, but the highest percentage of calories from fat overall. Studies have shown that the most fat calories and overall calories are burned by interval training—bursts of higher intensity activity, interspersed with a slightly lower level, recovery activity. In training terms, you move from a 65% intensity level to a peak 95% effort and back to 65%. Alpine environments naturally have this advantage, and you can and must replicate it if you want to see outstanding results.

Do the Math

To better understand my point, follow my math. Let's say we have a 150-pound person riding a stationary bike for 30 minutes. Going from 65% intensity to 95% and back to 65% can burn 173 calories, of which 50 calories come from fat. Keep in mind that it is your training intensity that matters. My maximum heart rate might be 185 beats per minute, while yours might be 160. Age has nothing to do with your maximum heart rate. An older person in her 50s who works out intensely several times per week can have a better aerobic capacity than a sedentary 20-year-old.

How do you determine your maximum heart rate? It depends more on your training experience and capacity. Hence, the formula of 220 minus age multiplied by intensity percentage does not apply and can be very misleading because two 55-year-olds, one active her entire life and the other always sedentary, would have the same intensity levels. Hence, the same calculation for both individuals gives you the same numbers for intensity levels to follow; so, it cannot be trusted.

You burn the most fat through the 65–95–65 system. When the same person performs true interval training for 30 minutes and changes the intensity level of her workout from 65% to 95% and back to 65%, she'll burn 173 calories, of which 50 calories could be from fat. Through this training, you're able to train both energy systems, aerobic and anaerobic, to take advantage of the benefit of burning off the most calories. This is true interval training and the basis for my Alpine Weight Loss Program. These workouts bring results, and if you don't feel like you're challenged and tired after those workouts, you only performed a medium-intensity workout and are not burning the most fat calories possible.

The **Alpine Aerobics Solution** follows the interval approach, which naturally occurs in the mountains. It naturally burns not only more calories and fat but also increases your motivation, endurance, and metabolism. You'll also improve your cardiovascular capacity. Research indicates that high-intensity training not only burns more fat more efficiently but also speeds up your metabolism long after your workout is completed. This is exactly what you want.

Mountains, Hills and Valleys: Your Personal Program

Dropping one, two or even three dress sizes can be done. For easy implementation there are three levels that I want you to accomplish. Once a week, do one Mountain Program, one Hill Program, and one Valley Program. That would make 3 aerobics programs per week. Each of them challenges you in different ways.

The Mountain Program. This program should be the most challenging for you. Think about a steep mountain that you need to walk up. Then go downhill and walk up another mountain. You can also jog, run, or bike this mountain. Just do it. Concentrate on overcoming the highest peak in order to get to the other side. This would be the 65-95-65 training approach. As you know by now, this approach burns not just the most fat calories but the highest total calories also. Your mountain can be created on a bike by increasing the resistance to climb the mountain. Create a mountain while walking by speeding up or finding hills to walk up at a brisk pace. Take the same approach while jogging or running. If you want to accomplish this in a gym, then use the treadmill and increase the incline and the speed. Near or around your home you can simply use an uphill driveway, stairs, or a bench that you step up and down on.

The Hill Program. We Alpine folks distinguish between mountains and hills. Hills are much smaller and flatter on the top. Hence, you don't have the high peaks to overcome. Rather you can manage to comfortably walk, jog, run, or bike up a hill with 85% intensity level throughout. The inclines are not as steep and not as long; they're short and manageable. But you will come to the point where you are out of breath.

The Valley Program. This is the easiest of all. Valleys are flat and do not have an incline; they give you the time to recover from the previous day's workout. With this program, you can walk, jog, run, or bike. Now here is a special trick for you. You can achieve the results of the Mountain Program within a Valley Program. How? Vary your speed of walking, jogging, running, and biking to create high peaks. Use speed walking, sprinting, or bike racing to create mountains to overcome, then recover in a flat environment—your valley.

Caution! If you are a beginner, stick to a Valley Program. When you have exercised more then 3 months, you can progress to the Hill Program and the Mountain Program. Don't get stuck in the Valley Program. In the Alps, individuals have no choice but to do the Mountain Program. Hence, they obtain the best results. If you expect to see the same results, increase your Mountain Program to 2 times per week and do the Valley or Hill Program only once a week.

Here is a 5-week sample program:

First Week: Tuesday: Hill Program; Thursday: Mountain Program; Saturday: Valley Program.

Second Week: Tuesday: Mountain Program; Thursday: Hill Program; Saturday: Valley Program.

Third Week: Tuesday: Valley Program; Thursday: Valley Program; Saturday: Mountain Program.

Fourth Week: Tuesday: Hill Program; Thursday: Valley Program; Saturday: Mountain Program.

Fifth Week: Tuesday: Mountain Program; Thursday: Valley Program; Saturday: Mountain Program.

Your Intensity Levels

For some, the challenge might arise after 10 minutes and for others, after 30 minutes into your Alpine Aerobics Program. For some, no challenge will arise in the Valley Program, but then challenge will arise in the Mountain Program. We are individuals with different priorities and genetics. It doesn't matter where you are currently. This program changes all the time. This program is about building up to reach your peaks (95% intensity intervals) and to look your best. We all have this ability if we choose to do it. And Alpine folks can't choose to do it.

1
2
3
4
5
6
7
8
9
10
11

They have to do it in order to be able to reach their neighbor just up the hill.

If you are new to cardio activity, start small. Start with 10 minutes, increase by 15 minutes until you're doing 30 minutes (longer if you wish and can) in the Valley, the Hill, and the Mountain Programs. Build up to it and enjoy the process of creating an efficient and youthful body again.

This program is dynamic instead of static. It should not be the same thing over and over. If you're not seeing results, it may be that you're not truly pushing yourself. Focus on how quickly and how steep a mountain you plan to conquer. There are so many different mountains and hills. Create them yourself in your own environment. For example, you might start with walking, then move into jogging, and drop back to a walk again. Or run, sprint, and run again. The point here is that you change your program each time—a bored body will not improve.

How do you know you are achieving the best results? Sweat. When your body temperature rises, your body needs to cool itself. We do this through our sweat when our body temperature rises because of muscle activity. Mountain Programs need to make you sweat. Otherwise you are not creating the intensity you need to burn the most calories and fat calories overall. Another indication is that you are getting slightly out of breath. Bravo! You have accomplished your goal.

Worksheet 9

Your current cardio program can move you forward or hold you back. Let's find out which is happening with you. During your cardio activity, do you flip through magazines, read a book, watch TV, or just move? Write down what kind of activity you do as your current Valley Program.

Your current Valley Program:

....

....

....

....

....

....

....

Did you catch yourself doing the same thing over and over again? Or perhaps not at all? Even so, you can start with your own Mountain Program once per week—it's as simple as speeding up the activity that you are performing, then recovering, and repeating it over and over again. Come up with 5 ways you could implement your own Mountain Program:

....

....

....

....

....

....

....

1
2
3
4
5
6
7
8
9
10
11

ALPINE
WEIGHT LOSS
SECRETS

12 Ways to Get the Alpine Advantage at Home

Personal Alpine environments for your Mountain Program can be created anywhere. In the desert, in pools, or just at home. Here are 12 ways to reach the 95% intensity peaks in 60 seconds or less:

1. **Mountain Knee Highs** – Sprint in place. Move your arms while you bring your knees up to hip height. Increase the intensity of this move by doing it while jumping rope.

2. **Chasing the Rabbit** – Place yourself in a push-up position on the floor. If you are on a wood, tile, or other slippery surface, place a towel under each foot. If carpet is your floor covering, then use paper plates or plastic bags under your feet. Bend your knees one at a time, bringing first your right then your left knee quickly toward to your chest. As you bend one knee in, straighten the other leg back out again.

3. **Brisk Hill Hike** – Walk or run up a flight of stairs. Change from single stairs to taking them 2 at a time.

4. **Bike the Alps** – Pedal as fast as you can up an incline; go faster if the incline isn't steep.

5. **Push the Tree** – Place your hands against a wall at about shoulder-height. Pretend you are able to push through the wall by performing the Mountain Knee Highs—quickly bringing your knees up and back to the floor.

6. **Over the Tree Trunk** – Use a box or a step (between 5 and 20 inches high). Bring one leg on the box, push yourself up, and land on the other side of the box with the other leg. Quickly repeat this motion. When you feel comfortable, add your hands by bringing them up and down when you push over the box.

7. **Run in the Fields** – Many families have a trampoline in the back garden for their children. Use them for your peaks by simply placing yourself in the middle of the trampoline and running in place with knee highs.

8. **Jump over the River** – Place a jump rope on the floor (a piece of string or a rolled up towel will also work). Jump or step from side to side over the rope while keeping both legs together. If possible, bring your knees up when you jump or step over the line.

ALPINE
WEIGHT LOSS
SECRETS

9   **Farmer's Walk/Run –** Take 2 heavy objects in your hands. Mark 2 points that are about 20 yards apart. Then walk or run briskly from one side to the other side while keeping your body upright. Some individuals will reach their peak by increasing only 10 pounds and some, 50 pounds.

10   **Chase the Deer –** Use the jump rope for this one. Start by jumping with both legs. When you feel comfortable, change to a quick jump rope run by increasing the speed of the jump rope. This is something to work up to. In case of existing knee pain, please check in with your doctor.

11   **Speed in Place –** Stay in place and move your feet 1 inch off the floor one at a time. Think you are moving as fast as you can but without actually moving forward. (Jennifer Beal in the movie Flash Dance performs it very well.) Then slow down and recover again.

12   **Race Your Kids –** Ever challenged your children physically? No? Try sprinting against them. (Of course let them sprint, and you can speed walk if this is what you can do comfortably.) Or go after a ball. Create 2 teams and compete against each other. Play tag. Be creative with them.

Remember this program is not static. Build up from the Valley to the Hill and finally to the Mountain Program. When you execute the Mountain Program start with one 95% peak level, add on a second, a third, and so forth. You can start first with 10 seconds, then 30 seconds, and build up to 60 seconds. When you get used to 60 seconds at 95% peak levels, increase to 120 second peaks. Try the different peak exercises as listed above. Keep it fun, challenging, and interesting.

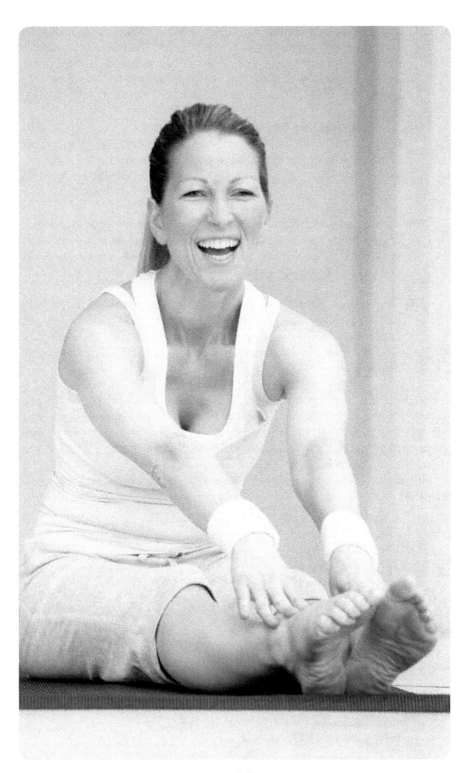

ALPINE
WEIGHT LOSS
SECRETS

Chapter 7

TRAIN YOURSELF "JUNG" [YOUNG]

Live Strong: Body Strength Training

You may not have grown up in a little village in Austria, but I'm guessing you, like most kids, pulled, pushed, twisted, walked, jumped, crawled, and sprinted without ever thinking about it, just as we still do in the Alps. Hopefully you were constantly running around, riding your bicycle, chasing after your friends, and automatically had more energy, tone, and muscle activation.

We are designed to walk, sprint, lunge, squat, bend, pull, push, and twist. As adults, many of us need to relearn how to run, sprint, jump, do push-ups, or twist. These are the basics of day-to-day living in the village and are the basics of any exercise program.

In the farming village where I grew up, there was almost always a physical goal or objective—either to cut the grass, feed the animals, or bring the harvest in as quickly as possible. We all helped to pick the grapes in the fall, pulling out the potatoes, beets, and carrots, and throwing the hay bales (at least 10 to 20 pounds each) on trucks to get them to the market. Was there a difference between what men and women did? No, everybody helped. And believe it or not, we youngsters often got fatigued much faster than the older and more experienced adults.

Now, some years later, living in the United States, I'm as active as ever. But what's happened around me? Everybody's going to gyms, which have become the new town square; the gym is now a hangout place without any physical goal besides talking with acquaintances. I see people standing around without an agenda or any kind of cohesive program. They read a book or magazine on the treadmill, talk on their cell phones, or just block out their brain by watching TV while working out. Or they go from dinner to the movies or theater; from home to the office; or from the office to the gym.

The results speak for themselves. Their bodies look the same, sometimes even worse, from year to year. Back home, the routines constantly changed as seasons changed. In the gym, the routines are often frozen in time.

The Alpine Longevity Strength Program will help you maintain your muscular system, skeletal system, lymphatic system, and immune system at an optimum performance level, so you stay young and agile and just as youthful and slender as Alpine villagers do.

Here's the idea: pulling up beetroots as a kid taught me that one beet might be more difficult to pull out than another. Sometimes we managed to get more work done in an hour and sometimes we did less. Our bodies quickly adapted to our activity level and we became stronger and leaner. By the end of the summer we all had very athletic-looking bodies. The same can be accomplished by implementing this Longevity Strength Program.

The Alpine Longevity Strength Program

Work in the garden or the field is never the same. Your program shouldn't be either. The Longevity Strength Program will help you connect with your most basic movement patterns that all of us were designed to do every day to stay in shape, strong, agile, and defined. These are the movements my neighbors did every day on the farm and in their gardens. And in these movements are all the primal movement patterns. And best of all you don't need a gym to perform them. You can do them right in your home, in your yard, your park, or when traveling.

The Longevity Strength Program moves target your arms, legs, and midsection with the least amount of impact to protect your joints. Just for fun, I have given you the garden or farm equivalent for each move. That will make them much more memorable, won't it?

ALPINE
WEIGHT LOSS
SECRETS

You need a tube (rubber band or weights if you have them already), a towel, and yourself.

Upper Body:

Milking the Cows – Triceps

1. Level 1 – Triceps extensions

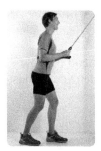 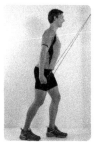

Place the tube over the door and take both ends in your hands.
Position the elbows at 90 degrees close to the body and implement the AAEs.
Pull the band down until your arms are straight. Return to starting position and repeat. If you are outside, perform the triceps dips as described below.

2. Level 2 – Triceps extensions, single arm

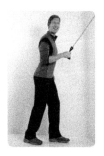 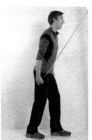

Place the tube over the door and take both ends in one hand.
Position the elbow at 90 degrees close to the body and implement the AAEs.
Pull the band down till your arm is straight only on the right side. Repeat on the right side before you change to the left side. Make it more challenging by shortening the band on the side of movement.

3. Level 3 – Triceps dips

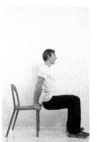 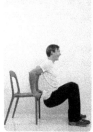

Sit on a chair, sofa, or bench and place your hands next to your body.
Lift your body up off the front edge of the seat and lower yourself in front of it. Keep the scapular activation (between the shoulders) and only go as far down as you feel comfortable.
Push yourself up again and repeat.

ALPINE
WEIGHT LOSS
SECRETS

1
2
3
4
5
6
7
8
9
10
11

Upper Body:

Picking the Pumpkins – Biceps

1. Level 1 – Biceps curls, both arms

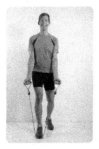 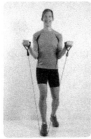

Stand with your right leg on the middle of the band while holding both ends of the band with your palms facing up. Your left leg stays back.
Pull your hands up until they're 5 inches away from the shoulders. Focus on keeping your shoulders in place.
Release the tension of the band by slowly straightening your arms to bring your hands to the starting position. Repeat.

2. Level 2 – Biceps curls, single arm

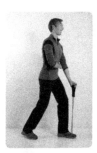 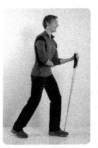

Stand with your right leg on the middle of the band while holding one end of the band with your palm facing up. Your left leg stays back.
Pull your right hand up only until 5 inches away from the shoulders. If you like, you can take both handlebars in one hand to increase the resistance.
Release the tension of the band by slowly straightening your arm to bring your right hand to the starting position and repeat.

Complete the repetitions and change to the other side.

3. Level 3 – Biceps curls

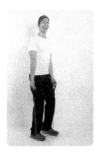 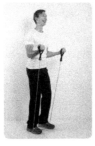

Stand with both legs on the middle of the band while holding both ends of the band with your palms facing up. Keep a wide stance so that you see the band between your legs. This will increase your resistance to make this a level 3 movement.
Pull your hands up until they're 5 inches away from the shoulders. Focus on keeping your shoulders in place; don't curl them into the band.

Release the tension of the band by slowly straightening your arms to bring your hands to the starting position. Repeat.

Upper Body:

Throwing the Pumpkin – Shoulder

1. Level 1 – Overhead presses, single arm

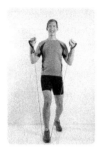 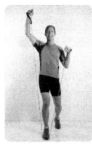

Hold both handles of an exercise band in your hands and place one foot in the center of the band.
Place both hands next to your shoulders.
Push up the right hand, straightening your arm overhead, and lower back to starting position. Repeat all repetitions before changing to the left side.

2. Level 2 – Overhead presses together

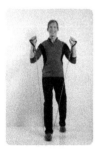 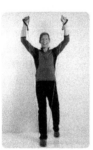

Hold both handles of an exercise tube in your hands and stand on the band. Both legs on the band will make it harder. One leg on the band will make it easier.
Place your hands next to the shoulders with your palms facing forward.
Push up the band toward the ceiling, straightening your arms overhead. Lower back to starting position and repeat.

3. Level 3 – Lateral lifts into overhead presses

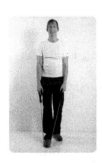 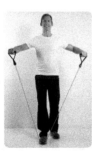

Step your right leg on the band. Hold the handles in each hand.
Place your hands next to your hips. Keeping arms straight, raise arms in front of chest, until your hands are level with shoulders (or slightly below them).
Lower your arms back to starting position and repeat.

1
2
3
4
5
6
7
8
9
10
11

Upper Body:

Picking the Weeds – Lateral pulls (back)

1. Level 1 – Cross pulls

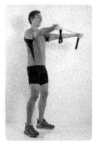 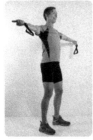

Hold the band at chest height with straight arms. Your palms should face up and your thumbs should point back (you can do this while standing or sitting; keep your abdominals engaged throughout the move).
Pull back the band keeping arms straight until the band touches the chest. Avoid letting your shoulders rise toward the ears.
Release the tension and let the arms come together again to the starting position. Repeat.

2. Level 2 – Lat pulls

Sit on the floor and extend both legs in front of you (keep your legs slightly bent). Wrap the tube around both feet, holding both ends in your hands palms facing in.
Straighten your back and bend your elbows. Pull your hands toward the sides of your body, at about belly button level.
Bring back the arms to the starting position and repeat.

3. Level 3 – Lat pulls, single arm

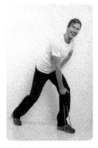 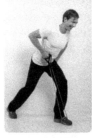

Place yourself into a standing lunge position (right leg in front).
Step on the tube with your right leg while you hold both ends of the tube in your left hand.
Pull the band toward the mid-body with your left arm; pause and then slowly straighten your arm to the starting position.
Repeat all repetitions before changing to the left side.

Upper Body:

Pushing the Sheep – Push-ups (chest)

1. Level 1 – Push-ups against the wall

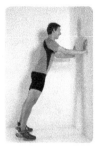 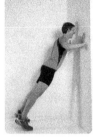

Stand in front of the wall and place your hands at shoulder level in front of you against the wall.
Lower your body by bending the arms toward the wall.
Push back into the starting position and repeat.

2. Level 2 – Push-ups on your knees

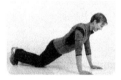 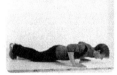

Kneel on the floor. Place your hands directly under your shoulders and activate the abdominals.
Lower your body toward the floor by bending your arms. Maintain the scapular activation by pressing shoulder blades toward the heels.
Push back into the starting position and repeat.

3. Level 3 – Push-ups from the toes

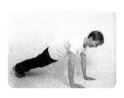 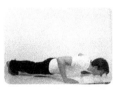

Kneel on the floor and place your hands under the shoulders.
Lift up your knees and hold this position from your toes. Activate the abdominals.
Lower your chest toward the floor and push back into the starting position again. Repeat.

ALPINE
WEIGHT LOSS
SECRETS

Lower Body:

Pulling up the Beets – squats (legs)

1. Level 1 – Squats over the chair

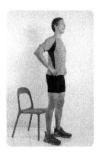 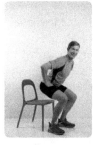

Stand in front of a chair. Implement the AAEs.

Push your bottom back while you bend your knees and maintain the activation in the abdominals.

Lower yourself until your bottom touches the chair and immediately stand back up into the starting position again. Repeat.

2. Level 2 – Assisted deep leg squats

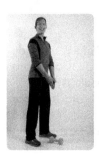 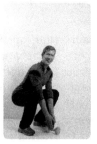

Stand between a doorframe and implement the AAEs. Place your hands on the side of the doorframe for support and balance.

Push your bottom toward the back and lean backward.

Bend your legs and lower yourself into a deep squat until hips touch the heels. You may need to build up to this level; start by coming down only as far as you feel comfortable doing. When you feel comfortable, substitute the doorframe with a dumbbell as shown. Aim to touch the dumbbell and stand up.

3. Level 3 – Deep leg squats

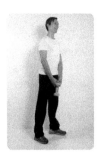 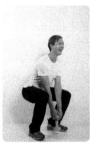

Stand upright and implement the AAEs (feel free to stay in the doorframe).

Bend your legs and push your bottom behind you while activating the transverse abdominal.

Lower your hips to your heels without holding on. Implement the Kegels to stand up to the starting position. Repeat. **TIP:** add on resistance with dumbbells; holding a weight in both hands or next to your hips or up by your shoulders

ALPINE
WEIGHT LOSS
SECRETS

Lower Body:

Skating the Creek – Lunges (legs)

1. Level 1 – Single leg standing lunges

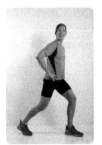 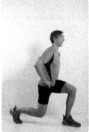

Place your right leg in front of you with your left leg back and bring your hands to your hips.

Activate through the AAEs and bend your knees to lower your hips toward the floor until your back knee is approximately is 8-10 inches off floor.

Straighten your legs again to the starting position. Repeat all repetitions on one side before you change to the other side.

2. Level 2 – Single leg step back

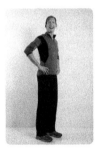 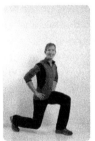

Stand with both feet together and place your hands on your hips.

Step back with your right leg into the lunge position as described above.

Lean your torso slightly forward to maintain the weight on the left leg and step back to the starting position. Do all repetitions with the same leg before changing to the other side.

3. Level 3 – Single leg slide back (You need a towel)

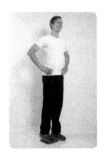 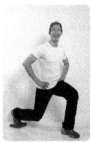

Stand with both feet together. Place your hands to your hips and rest your right foot on a towel on a slippery surface (such as a wood or tile floor).

Slide your right leg (on the towel) back while you bend your left leg into a lunge. Only slide as far back as you can and stay stable.

Slide forward to the starting position and repeat. Switch legs and repeat.

1
2
3
4
5
6
7
8
9
10
11

Lower Body:

Pushing the Cart – Gluteus and quadriceps (legs)

1. Level 1 – Pushing the wall (both legs pushing)

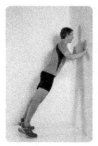 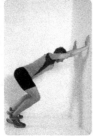

Place both hands on the wall (use a tree when you are outdoors) and position your feet so that your body is in a 50-degree angle to the floor/ground.
Bend your legs. Stick your bottom to the back. (Imagine you are performing a squat.)
Straighten the legs and try to move the wall/tree away. Repeat.

2. Level 2 – Pushing the wall (one-leg pushes)

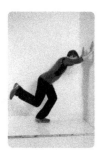 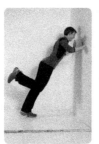

Place both hands on the wall (use a tree when you are outdoors) and position your feet away from the wall/tree so that you're at a 50-degree angle to the floor/ground.
Lift up one leg and bend the standing leg. Stick you bottom to the back. (Imagine you are per-forming a single leg squat.)
Straighten the standing leg and try to move the wall/tree away while the opposite leg stays off the ground. Repeat.

3. Level 3 – Pushing the floor (You need a towel)

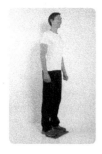

Stand on a wooden or tile floor on a towel. Position your feet shoulder-width apart on a towel. (Substitute a plastic bag for the towel if you have a carpet.) Keep arms by your sides.
Bend your legs and bring your hands on the floor. Push your legs and feet out till you are in a push-up position.
Pull the legs back in using your abdominals muscles and stand up. Repeat.

Lower Body:

Lifting the Sheep – Calf raises (calves)

1. Level 1 – Heel raises

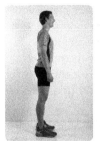 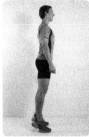

Find a step and stand with the balls of both feet on the edge of the step.
Lower the heels toward the floor.
Raise your body again by pushing the toes into the step. Practice your posture with this movement.

2. Level 2 – Single-leg heel raises

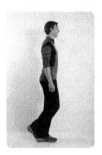 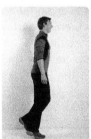

Stand on a step with the balls of both feet on the edge of the step.
Cross your right leg behind your left heel so that you are only standing on one leg.
Lower the heel toward the floor and push back up again. Finish repetitions on one side before changing to the other side.

3. Level 3 – Heel raises with resistance

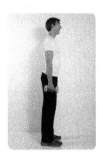 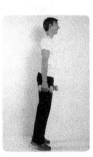

Execute the same movement as before and add additional resistance by holding a barbell or any kind of other weight such as a gallon container of water.

1
2
3
4
5
6
7
8
9
10
11

Lower Body:

Kicking the Horse – Bottom

1. Level 1 – Single leg extensions

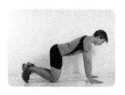 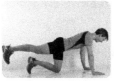

Kneel on the floor and place your hands under the shoulders. Pull in your stomach and maintain the activation throughout the movement.

Extend the right leg behind you, keeping the foot flexed (toes pulled toward you). Do not raise your heel higher than your bottom.

Bend the leg so that the knee makes a right angle and the sole of your foot is pointing up. Straighten back to the starting position and repeat. Finish the repetitions on one side before changing to the next.

2. Level 2 – Single leg extensions with tube

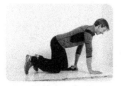 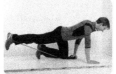

Kneel on the floor and place your hands under the shoulders. Position the tube around the right foot and secure the end of the tube with your opposite knee by kneeling on it. Or hold the handles with your hand if you like.

Extend the right leg until the leg is straight. Keep your foot flexed and avoid raising your heel higher than your bottom.

Bring back the leg to the starting position and repeat. Finish the repetitions on one side before changing to the next.

3. Level 3 – Single leg extensions with tube

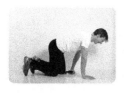 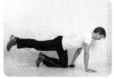

Kneel on the floor and place your hands under the shoulders. Position the tube around the right foot and secure the end of the tube with your opposite knee by kneeling on it. Or hold the handle with your hand if you like.

Extend the right leg until the leg is straight. Keep your foot flexed and avoid raising your heel higher than your bottom.

Bring back the leg to the starting position and repeat. To make it a level 3 exercises shorten the tube or use a more difficult tube. Finish the repetitions on one side before changing to the next.

ALPINE
WEIGHT LOSS
SECRETS

Lower Body:

Building a Bridge – Hamstrings

1. Level 1 – Leg bridge

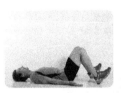 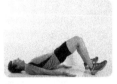

Lie on your back and bend your legs so your feet are flat on the floor. Activate your abdominals.
Push up your bottom while pressing your heels into the floor. Clench the cheeks of your bottom together.
Avoid arching your back and keep your legs hip-width apart.
Lower your bottom to the starting position and repeat.

2. Level 2 – Single leg bridge

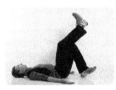 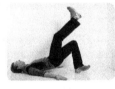

Lie on your back and keep your legs bent (same as before).
Lift up your bottom and hold this position without arching your back. Raise your right leg toward the ceiling.
Lower your bottom again and push back up again while the right leg stays up. Finish the repetitions on one side before changing to the next.

3. Level 3 – Single leg slide (You need a towel)

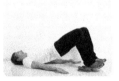 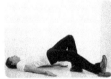

Lie on your back, bend your legs, and place 2 towels under your feet.
Lift up your bottom and slide your right leg forward while trying to keep your bottom up.
Slide your right leg back to the starting position while the left leg moves forward. Immediately change your legs again and repeat. Start with 10 seconds, then 20 seconds until you reach 30 seconds.

Mid-body:

Threshing the Fields – Transverse abdominus (abs)

1. Level 1 – Russian twists (legs down)

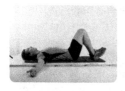 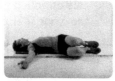

Lie on your back. Position arms at shoulder level on the floor. Bend your legs and keep your heels on the floor.

Move your knees toward the right side until legs are almost touching the floor. Only go as far as you can without lifting the opposite shoulder off the floor. Maintain the activation in your abdominals.

Move your knees back to the starting position and lower to the other side. Repeat.

2. Level 2 – Russian twists (bend 45 degrees)

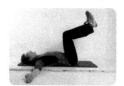 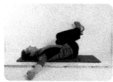

Lie on your back. Position arms at shoulder level on the floor. Bend both legs and lift your heels off the floor so that your knees form a 90-degree angle.

Move your knees toward the right side without changing the angle of your legs. Only lower as far as you can without lifting the opposite shoulder from the floor. Maintain the activation in your abdominals.

Lift your knees up to the starting position and lower to the other side. Repeat.

3. Level 3 – Russian twists (with weight)

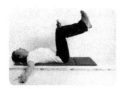 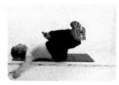

Lie on your back. Lift both legs off the floor so that knees form a 90-degree angle. Position arms to shoulder level on floor. Place a weight between your knees.

Lower your legs toward the right side by keeping legs straight. Only lower as far as you can without lifting the opposite shoulder from the floor. Maintain the activation in your abdominals.

Raise your legs back up to the starting position and lower to the other side. Repeat.

Lower Body:

Holding the Bridge – Core strength (abs)

1. Level 1 – Plank holding from your knees

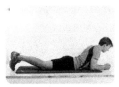 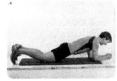

Kneel on the floor and place your elbows under the shoulders.

Position your body so that your knees align with your hips, shoulders, and head. Press hips up off the floor.

Activate the abdominals and hold this position for 10 seconds, 20 seconds. Build up to holding for 60 seconds.

2. Level 2 – Plank holding from your toes

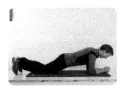 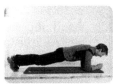

Kneel on the floor and place your elbows under the shoulders.

Position your body so that your hips align with your shoulders and knees while the knees are on the floor. Press hips up off the floor.

Lift up the knees and hold this position for 10 seconds. Build up 10 seconds at a time until you can hold the position for 60 seconds.

3. Level 3 – Plank holding, single leg

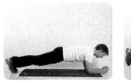 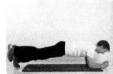

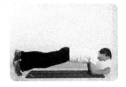

Start out as above in a plank position.

Lift up your right leg 1 inch off the floor and hold this position for 10 seconds.

Lower the right leg and lift up the left leg and hold this position for 10 seconds. Repeat up to 6 repetitions on each side.

Mid-body:

Holding the Bridge Sideways – Obliques

1. Level 1 – Lateral plank (knees down)

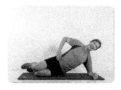 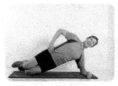

Place yourself on your side and position the elbow under the shoulder.
Bend both legs and flex your feet (toes to you).
Lift up your hip and hold this position for 10 seconds. Switch sides and repeat 3 times.

2. Level 2 –Lateral plank (one knee up)

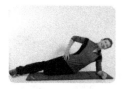 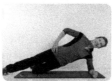

Place yourself sideways on the floor. Position the elbow under the shoulder.
Bend your bottom leg behind you while you keep the top leg extended with the foot on the floor.
Lift up your hip from the floor, pressing down with the top leg. Be sure to keep your foot, knee, and hip aligned. Lower to starting position and repeat. Do all repetitions on one side before switching to the other side.

3. Level 3 – Lateral plank (both knees up)

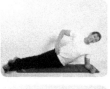 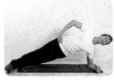
 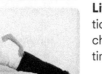

Place yourself on your side and position the elbow under the shoulder.
Straighten both legs and flex your feet (toes to you).
Lift up your hip and hold this position. Hold for 10 counts before you change to the other side. Repeat 3 times.

Lower Body:

Hunting with the Bird Dog – Back extensions

1. Level 1 – Bird dog (kneeling)

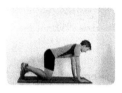 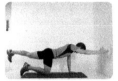

Kneel on the floor with your hands under the shoulders and your knees under your hips.

Pull in your stomach toward your spine (AAEs). Lift up the right knee and the left arm off the floor.

Extend the arm and leg until level with the body (not higher). Lower back to starting position. Switch sides and repeat.

2. Level 2 – Bird dog (lying)

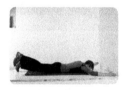 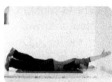

Lie on your stomach on the floor. Extend both arms overhead in a V position. Turn your thumbs toward the ceiling.

Lift up your right arm and left leg while keeping the forehead on the floor. Keep the stomach pulled toward the spine.

Lower your right arm and your left leg back to start. Switch sides and repeat.

3. Level 3 – Bird dog (whole body lifts)

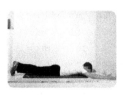 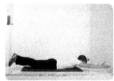

Lie on your stomach on the floor. Extend your arms in front of you into a V position. Turn your thumbs toward the ceiling.

Lift up both arms, both legs, and your head while you keep your stomach pulled toward the spine. Do not hyperextend (increased arch).

Lower your hands and legs back to starting position and repeat.

1
2
3
4
5
6
7
8
9
10
11

Lower Body:

Walking the Farmers Walk – Posture

1. Level 1 – Walk

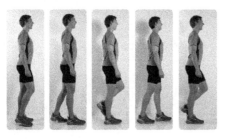

Stand upright, arms at your sides, and press your shoulder blades down. Keep your chin level to the floor. (A quick check: Place a fist on the top of your breastbone; your chin should touch the top of your fist.)

Activate the midsection (transverse abdominus) and start walking approximately 20 yards. Avoid swinging your hips from side to side. Stay stable.

Turn around and walk another 20 yards. Repeat 4 times.

2. Level 2 – Walk with resistance

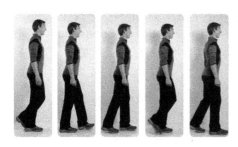

Stand upright, press your shoulder blades down, and keep the chin level to the floor. Optional: hold 2 gallon water jugs with straight arms next to your body (you can substitute weights).

Activate the midsection (transverse abdominus) and start walking approximately 20 yards. Avoid swinging your hips from side to side. Stay stable.

Turn around and walk another 20 yards. Repeat 4 times.

3. Level 3 – Run with resistance

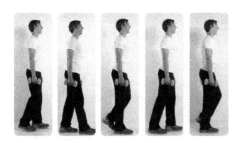

Stand upright, press your shoulder blades down, and keep your chin level to the floor. Hold 2 gallon water jugs with straight arms next to your body (you can substitute weights).

Activate the midsection (transverse abdominus) and start running approximately 20 yards. Avoid swinging your hips from side to side. Stay stable.

Turn around and run another 20 yards. Repeat 4 times.

This might be a lot to digest. Also I am aware that a book is much harder to carry than a single page with your program. I also know everyone learns differently. Some learn through auditory means, some learn by reading, and some learn by observing.

That's why I designed workout templates for you that you can print and carry with you. You will see the images and names of the exercise. Going outdoors will be a pleasure and a change of pace.

Staying active during travel will be easy. Staying committed at home will be a breeze. And you will be able to follow your program knowing exactly what to do.

**Go to www.AlpineWeightLossSecrets.com/BookBonusLogIn.html
I will send you your free workout sheets and other tools to follow
right over.**

How to Implement the Alpine Longevity Strength Program

Split up your **Alpine Longevity Strength Program** into upper body and mid-body for one session, then the lower body and mid-body the second work-out, and the full body routine the third day. For example, the best plan would be to work out every Monday, Wednesday, and Friday. For additional variety, start out the first week with the upper body, the next week with your lower body, and the following week with your full body program. I guarantee you won't be bored with this approach!

How long will it take? When you move once through each section (upper, lower, or mid-body), it will not take longer than 5 to 7 minutes for the single set. Your goal will be to build up to a second set and possibly a third. Here is your 3-week sample program:

First Week: Monday: Upper and Mid-Body Program; Wednesday: Lower and Mid-Body Program; Friday: Upper, Lower, and Mid-Body Program (Combined, this is referred to as the Full Body Program.)

Second Week: Monday: Full Body Program; Wednesday: Upper and Mid-Body Program; Friday: Lower and Mid-Body Program

Third Week: Monday: Lower and Mid-Body Program; Wednesday: Upper and Mid-Body Program; Friday: Full Body Program

Time commitment is always an issue. Yes, it can be a challenge when there are schedules or appointments to keep. Make it interesting and make it work for you. Get more bang for your buck by just doing one section of the program every second day, which will not take longer than 5 to 7 minutes at the most. Monday follow the Upper Body Program, Wednesday the Lower Body Program, and Friday the Mid-Body Program.

Here is your 3-week sample program:

First Week:
Monday: Upper Body Program;
Wednesday: Lower Body Program;
Friday: Mid-Body Program

Second Week:
Monday: Lower Body Program;
Wednesday: Mid-Body Program;
Friday: Upper Body Program

Third Week:
Monday: Mid-Body Program;
Wednesday: Upper Body Program;
Friday: Lower Body Program

Remember, this program is not for heavy-duty bodybuilders and for gym rats. Rather, this is a program for individuals who want to stay active but don't want to go to the gym, and still want to see results in terms of body definition, weight loss, and looking younger naturally. This program is to accomplish long-lasting lifestyle changes. Perhaps you are wondering yourself if you need to work against resistance? Yes, you do, and you will.

5 Ways to Challenge Yourself: The 3R2S System

Variety and progression are built into this strength program. Level one is frankly best if you're just starting out with strength training. But don't underestimate the toughness involved in even a basic move. Holding a position (even with no weights and just your body weight) is challenging. Level 2 is for the advanced person, and level 3 is for the experienced person. Still, go back to some of the starter moves occasionally. Hold the move longer and really focus on form. Or challenge yourself using some of these strategies.

The Mix-It-Up 3R2S System

As a general rule, start with just the movement itself. This will give you time to familiarize yourself with the movement. Then implement the 3R2S system.

ALPINE
WEIGHT LOSS
SECRETS

First R: Resistance – Increase the resistance. You can do this by using either weights (in the form of dumbbells, barbells, rubber bands, or a medicine ball) or simply changing the position of your body.

Second R: Repetition – Vary your reps. Do 3 sets of an exercise: Start with 10 repetitions for the first set, then 15 for the next, and 20 repetitions for the final set. You may have to adjust the amount of resistance you're using, but this is a good way to develop muscle tone.

Third R: Rest – Accelerate your results. This is the level where you will see the most results by burning the most overall fat. Reduce your resting period from 90 seconds to 60, 30 to 15 seconds. And once every 2 weeks, you will not rest at all between any exercises.

First S: Speed – Pick up your speed. Create muscle definition and burn more calories. In my childhood, there were many times when the harvested wheat or vegetables needed to be brought in before the end of the day, especially before it started to rain. Speed was how we pushed ourselves to get it done. This level will help you to build your muscle tissue, increasing your intensity to peak points to create an agile, younger body. Instead of performing an exercise in 10 seconds, reduce it to 5 or 3 seconds. This will depend on your capability to maintain the form and control that you learned in the first level.

Second S: Sets – Build your endurance. Decrease the amount of rest between sets. This will help you to build your lactic acid threshold, which allows you to be active longer without getting tired during the day or during weekend activities. When you first try this, simply do an exercise once before you move to the next. When you feel confident of being able to increase your speed and resistance, try repeating an exercise up to 4 times consecutively. Why? Can you imagine just picking 1 beet per day to bring the harvest in?

The Shortcut Solution:
The Alpine Youngevity Fitness Program

By now you've realized that this is a 6-day program. Wahoo, isn't it great? So quick and so easy. Even so, many times you might run into time constraints due to the basic ins-and-outs of life. When time is tight (or you need to see results in a hurry), I suggest combining the **Alpine Aerobic Solution** with the **Alpine Longevity Strength Program**. Then it becomes the Alpine Youngevity Fitness Program. It mimics what individuals in Alpine environments do daily: A mix of cardiovascular training and daily strength training to stay on top of their environment.

In this combined program, it is best to start out with the *Alpine Aerobic Solution* followed by the *Alpine Longevity Strength Program*.

Sample Program 1:
As before, choose your Alpine Aerobic Solution Program.
Then rotate through the targeted body strength programs. For example:

Mountain Program and Upper Body Program;
Hill Program and Mid-Body Program;
Valley Program and Lower Body Program
(A word of caution: do not perform the Lower Body Program after the Mountain Program unless you are an in shape and trained.)

Sample Program 2:
In this plan, you add in more targeted strength moves after each Alpine Aerobic Solution session. For example:

Mountain Program first, followed by Upper Body and Mid-Body Program;
Hill Program first, followed by Lower Body and Mid-Body Program;
Valley Program first followed by Full Body Program

Do not jump into this program until you have had ample experience and training through Sample Program 1.)

Sample Program 3:
Kick your rear into gear! This is the program that achieves results fast if you have to get ready for a special event such as a wedding, reunion, emergency summer vacation, or last-minute adventure trips. Of course, you need to be able to execute the moves correctly and build up to this level.

Mountain Program first followed by Full Body Program;
Hill Program first followed by Full Body Program;
Valley Program first followed by Full Body Program;

Try These 6 Lifestyle Toners

Day-to-day activities contribute to the overall goal. They can keep you young, strong, and focused, as your mind will be occupied with doing little changes, and you'll achieve big results.

Road-test these 6 tips:

❶   **Pick up your day.** Once a day, pick something up heavier than 10 pounds, say a bag of cat litter or a small upholstered chair. But don't pick it up in just any old way. Start by bending your legs into a deep squat instead of bending from your back.

❷   **Use your body, not just your mind.** We have become knowledge workers, just working with our minds. Make an effort to train your body as you train your mind. With consistency. Be active at least 20 to 30 minutes per day. Little bursts of activity add up, so always take the stairs. Even climbing the escalator counts! Instead of your usual bus stop, walk to the next one, if possible.

❸   **Choose a green spot.** This might be a park, your back garden, or maybe a room or deck with a view of treetops. Perhaps a sky. This will be your go-to longevity spot for relaxation. Taking time to decompress is vital to staying young and avoiding burnout.

❹   **Set some speed control.** You've mastered a workout routine. Great, work with it. The next time you do it, change the speed, either to super slow from fast or from super slow to a controlled and faster movement.

❺   **Focus on progress.** End goals are important, but it's the journey–the progressive improvements—that you celebrate. The more often you acknowledge them, the more motivated you'll be to stay the course and get you to the end goal.

❻   **Track and measure.** Every 4 weeks measure yourself. Don't just weigh yourself. Use circumference and body fat measurements as well. Each of those measurements gives you indications of what is happening with your body. Weight is not the only measurement. How your clothes fit and how you look are all important.

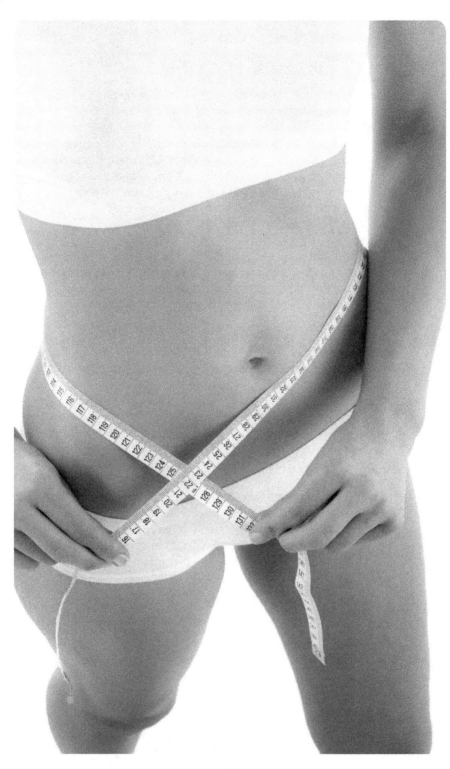

ALPINE
WEIGHT LOSS
SECRETS

Chapter 8

A FLAT BELLY – "SCHNELL" (FAST)!

Alpine Anti-bloat Plan

The Holy Grail of fitness for many of my clients is a flat, toned, trim abdomen (belly). So many clients come to me frustrated because, despite bunches of crunches, they still have a pot, a pooch, or a muffin top. As a trainer, I know that to shape and tone your belly, you really need a three-pronged approach: determination, nutrition, and activation.

Even the fitness industry did not always have it right—crunches were once touted as the number 1 strategy for flattening the stomach. The more you did the better. Infomercials really got us with this hoax. Think ab buster, ab rocker, and more. But only your wallet got flatter, and now that "miracle machine" is gathering dust in the corner. Extreme diets were the next cure for a flabby belly. There were plans to change the protein, carb, and fat ratios. Sometimes sugar was the culprit, alcohol, chemicals, and caffeine—you name it! In the quest for a get-flatter-faster food, exercise was just about forgotten. Now we know: for long-lasting changes and results you will need personal nutrition and exercise and determination.

As you have figured out by now, the Alpine Advantage is an approach that works with nutrition, activity, and your mental muscle to help you to achieve not only optimal health but optimal beauty and body.

Get Flatter Faster!

Let's face it—quick results are motivating. To sharpen your weight loss

ALPINE
WEIGHT LOSS
SECRETS

or toning focus and jump-start your body's restorative process, first flush your systems with fresh oxygen. Do this with activity in fresh air. You can do this right now. The trees give up oxygen in the evening and when walking to oxygenate your body, the evening is preferred. Second, cleanse your digestive and metabolic systems. One of the reasons why your belly does not get flatter can be because you have inflammation due to any ingredients that you are allergic to or food in your digestive track that does not move.

So, let us flatten your belly, clean out your internal garbage, get rid of bloating, and reduce inflammation. In two to three days, expect to have a flatter stomach and feel flooded with energy.

The 2-Day Alpine Cleansing Cure

The 2-day Alpine Cleansing Cure is done by juicing. The benefits of juicing have been appreciated for centuries. Juicing gives your digestive system—the stomach, intestines, pancreas, gallbladder, and liver—a rest. During this process, these organs (and their constituent cells) have the time to repair and get rid of waste. Your body gets an opportunity to put its energy into elimination, recovery, and healing. When you juice over a period of time, you consume fewer calories, so your liver converts its stored glycogen to readily available glucose and energy. During this process of detoxification, many clients say they experience a new clarity of mind and a pure feeling in their bodies.

Juicing and fasting are different. Fasting means you drink only water. With juicing, you still provide your body with nutrients from freshly squeezed vegetables. (In some cases, people add fruits, but in this plan there are no fruits in the first 14 days. Why? Read about the yeast issue in chapter 3: *Alpine Eating: Choose Tomatoes Not Potatoes.* When you fast, protein breakdown occurs and that is less likely to happen when juicing with vegetables and broth.

Timing is vital, and juicing should be limited to 1, 2, or, at most, 3 days. While experienced fasters can go as long as 40 days without foods under the proper supervision, there is no need to be this extreme. If getting enough protein and preventing tissue breakdown are concerns for you, then just supplement your juicing program with brown rice milk, soymilk, or spirulina (contains between 55% and 77% protein) to provide your body with amino acids. Keep your eyes on the prize: a bloat-free belly!

For 2 days, you will be drinking mostly liquids such as vegetable juices, teas, and water. These contain plenty of nutrients that are beneficial to your digestion and your sodium-potassium balance, which will help reduce swelling and body puffiness due to water retention. The third day is a transition day, designed to reintroduce solid foods.

Do not worry that you will not get enough nutrients during the days of juicing. On the contrary, you will receive vitamins, minerals, and enzymes in concentrated doses that will help your system function more efficiently. It is like giving your car the best gasoline available. You would have to eat a lot of vegetables to get the same amount of nutrients from drinking 3 to 4 vegetable juices per day.

Some people feel so comfortable with juicing during day 1 that they want to keep going. It is usually safe to continue for 2 or 3 days, but check with your medical practitioner before extending your juicing program, just to be safe. You will feel a sense of satisfaction and calmness and be energized in new ways. You can repeat the first 2-Day Plan every 2 weeks or if you simply feel you need to get back on track and refocus.

FREE RADICALS AND JUICING

If we talk about designing a younger you, more vital and energetic, we need to understand what free radicals are, what they do in your body, and how to get rid of them.

First, what are free radicals? They are unstable molecules that are damaging to cells. They are created by the normal processes of energy production, breathing, and solar radiation. Biological oxidation, the process of making energy, involves moving electrons, which are around the nucleus of an atom, from one oxygen molecule to the next. But sometimes an electron escapes. This free electron is called a free radical, and it can oxidize DNA, damage fat molecules traveling in the bloodstream, and set us up for heart disease, stroke, and premature aging. Antioxidants from fruits, vegetables, and supplementation may be one of the most effective ways to prevent cell damage and to slow down aging. They merge with the free radicals. Then the free radicals can be disarmed and weakened without doing any damage. This process occurs about 10,000 times in each cell per day.

To slow down aging, your job is to provide your body with sufficient antioxidants to get rid of free radicals safely without doing any damage to your cells and DNA. The Alpine Cleansing Cure is 1 simple strategy that you can do to provide your system with instant absorbable antioxidants while flattening your belly.

1
2
3
4
5
6
7
8
9
10
11

Your Beat-the-Bloat Plan

Drink only liquids for breakfast, snack 1, lunch, snack 2, and dinner for an entire day. Throughout the day, drink as much as you like from the following choices:

- Vegetable juice (8-ounce serving). Stick to these ingredients: lemon juice, carrots, beets, spinach, cucumber, celery, parsley, ginger, and cinnamon. Add a drop of extra virgin olive oil or pumpkin seed oil to prevent insulin surges with each juice meal. This will help stabilize your blood sugars and maintain energy throughout the day.
- Teas such as peppermint and chamomile. Also try fresh ginger cinnamon tea: use 5 slices of fresh ginger and 1 cinnamon stick; simmer for 20 minutes. Let it cool in the refrigerator and drink it with freshly squeezed lemon juice.
- Homemade chicken or vegetable broth.
- Plenty of plain water. (A squeeze of lemon in it is refreshing!)

2-Day Alpine Cleansing Cure Sample Menus

Day One

1 glass water with fresh lemon
Peppermint tea

Breakfast
Carrot, lemon

Snack 1
Carrot, lemon, beets

Lunch
Carrot, spinach, cucumber

Snack 2
Cucumber, celery, carrot

Dinner
Beets, parsley, carrot, cinnamon

Day Two

1 glass water with fresh lemon
Peppermint tea

Breakfast
Carrot, lemon, parsley

Snack 1
Cucumber, celery, carrot

Lunch
Spinach, beets, ginger

Snack 2
Cucumber, carrot, lemon

Dinner
Beets, parsley, carrot, cinnamon

TIP: Drink tea as a snack if you do not have access to juices

ALPINE
WEIGHT LOSS
SECRETS

Why these ingredients produce a flat belly

Why the strict list? Each of the ingredients recommend here has proven belly-flattening or anti-bloating benefits. Stick to my list and see results!

Lemons are a fat emulsifier, enhancing bile activity. Bile is produced by the liver and stored in the gall bladder; a little gland by the liver. By improving your bile level, you will accelerate weight loss and fat metabolism. You will also enjoy better digestion. The tartness of lemon juice also makes you feel fuller and more satisfied much sooner.

Carrots got a bad rap when the glycemic index was published. This index measures the increase of blood sugar after consumption of a food. The higher the insulin levels rise after the consumption of a food, the worse off you are in terms of weight loss. It is crazy. When you compare a candy bar to a carrot, the candy bar has a lower glycemic load. One of the reasons for this is that the candy bar has fat, which slows the rise in blood sugar. Fiber does the same thing; unfortunately, when you juice carrots, the fiber is removed. To counter this, just mix it with other vegetables (spinach, for example) and add a few drops of olive oil. Carrots are high in potassium, vitamin A, and alpha carotene. They also help to establish a beneficial potassium-to-sodium ratio [2:1] for weight loss.

Beets are a fantastic liver tonic. The liver is the Grand Central Station of toxins; any toxin that is ingested or produced in the body gets dumped here for cleansing and detoxification. As you lose fat, stored metals, pesticides, and hormones are released; the liver needs to filter those materials. Hence, it is very important to maintain a healthy and functioning liver during this process. Also, beets are high in iron, betaine, and folate. These last two work in synergy to reduce potential toxic levels of homocysteine, a naturally occurring amino acid that can be harmful to blood vessels, thereby contributing to the development of heart disease, stroke, dementia, and vascular diseases. Finally, beets are loaded with potassium. Use the leaves as well as the root when you juice because they are even higher in nutritional value than the root.

Spinach is a power green. Calorie for calorie, green leafy vegetables provide more nutrients than almost any other food on the planet. Unfortunately, spinach is also one of the vegetables most heavily sprayed with fertilizers and chemicals. That is why organically grown is best. Spinach is chockful of calcium, magnesium, and vitamins D and K. Vitamin K contains osteocalcin, which anchors calcium molecules inside the bone. It is also great for your brain. According to a study reported in the May 2005 issue of the Journal of Experimental Neurology, rats fed a diet enriched with spinach and blue-berries lost a lot fewer brain cells after a stroke and had a fuller recovery than rats that were not eating the spinach and blueberry-enriched diets. You cannot go wrong with spinach, and you will find spinach in almost every back garden in any little Alpine village.

1
2
3
4
5
6
7
8
9
10
11

Cucumbers are another Alpine garden staple, and they are easy to grow and low in calories. Because of their high water content, cucumbers are a natural for juicing. They are known as a very good natural diuretic. Some people suffer gastric difficulties with the seeds. If that is the case, just scrape the seeds out and use the rest.

Celery is very low in calories and is fantastic to fat-flush your system because of its high fiber content and high water content. It is terrific for appetite control as it is low on the glycemic index. There is also nutrition in the stalks too, such as silicon that can help renew joints, bones, arteries, and connective tissues. Celery also contains acetylenes, which have been shown to stop the growth of cancer cells.

Parsley may be small, but it is a potent diuretic, blood purifier, and blood vessel rejuvenator because of its high vitamin C, beta carotene, B12, chlorophyll, and essential fatty acid content. It is your leafy multivitamin!

Cinnamon is a typical Alpine spice. It helps to regulate your blood sugar, reduce bad cholesterol, and can help ease pain and stiffness in muscles and joints. It contains the phytochemicals eugenol and geraniol, which can fight candida (yeast) because of their antibacterial and antifungal activities. It also relieves gas, and its anti-inflammatory compounds can soothe menstrual discomfort. Why is cinnamon an Alpine spice when cinnamon's original heritage is Sri Lanka and China? If only I knew.

THE FRESH JUICE FIX

It is always best to drink freshly made juice. Remember: pasteurized = processed, which means fewer nutrients, no enzymes, and no light energy. If you do not have a juicer available, here are a few solutions:

• Make your own anti-bloat drink by grating a thumb-size piece of ginger and squeezing the juice from lemons. Combine in a pitcher of water, add ½ teaspoon ground cinnamon; stir, and it is ready to drink.

• Drink broth from freshly made chicken and vegetable soups only. (Only use the processed versions in an emergency.) No cream-based soup such as clam chowder or broccoli cream soup.

• Buy pasteurized juices such as Odwella and add the juice from 1 freshly squeezed lemon.

Ana: Jumping for Juicing!

Ana inquired about my program after a feature about it appeared on a very well-known online publication. At 5 feet 7 inches, this African American woman in her 30s had a fantastic sense of style and fashion. We met to chat and get to know each other. During our conversation, she admitted that she recently gained about 40 pounds, and that she felt disgusted about herself. Her new job had taken its toll, and she had no time for anything but work. But her wedding was 11 months away. She wanted to start to get her body back on track. After years playing sports, she had great fitness fundamentals and a solid foundation that we could work with. But she wanted to have results fast to jump-start the process of transformation.

After the review of her food log, her downfalls were clear. Lunch was deli foods; diet sodas, chocolates, and chips were the snacks of choice. She was a typical type A personality who liked to get things done when she put her mind to it. That is why she opted for the 2-Day Alpine Cleansing Cure. When I saw her on the third day for her workout, I noticed a big change in her energy; even her belly was noticeably flatter. Her attitude had changed as well. As she later explained to me, her relationship with food had changed. She no longer lived to eat, but ate to live, choosing to nourish her body with the freshest and best foods possible. It just made her feel more alive, she said.

After continuing with the follow-up program, Ana went from 186 pounds to 142 pounds. Her body fat percentage dropped from 39.9% to 25.5%, and her waist and hip measurements from 33/42 to 26/33—all in just 20 weeks! Needless to say, she accomplished her goal and credits the quick and visible results from the 2-Day Alpine Cleansing Cure as the "easy pass" on her road to success.

12 Flat Belly Tips

After the two-day program, it is best to gradually introduce solid food again. Here are some more guidelines for shopping and putting together satisfying menus and meals.

Carbohydrates: Eat whole grains only: brown rice, oats, rye, quinoa, amaranth, millet, buckwheat, barley, and whole wheat. They are packed with fiber and keep your insulin levels up, which helps you to stay mentally alert and provides you with sustained energy. No white pasta, pastry, or breads containing yeast and/or sugar. Belly bloating can also result from mild gluten intolerance; your body cannot digest gluten, and an inflammatory response may occur. To be on the safe side, start out with gluten-free grains such as millet, brown rice, wild rice, and cornmeal (not a grain). If you think you have gluten intolerance, get tested by your doctor.

Protein: Eat plenty of organic white chicken or turkey, fresh cold-water and salt-water fish, and tofu. No cured, smoked, barbecued, pickled, fatty, or red meats. Stay away from red meat for now because it slows down your digestion transition time. The last thing you want right now is anything that slows you down, especially when it comes to your energy levels.

Dairy: Eat low or nonfat plain yogurt, which helps replenish the healthy bacteria in your digestive system. If you are lactose intolerant, substitute rice milk or brown rice milk for cow's milk in recipes. But in general, avoid dairy products during the after program aside from low or nonfat plain yogurt.

Oils: Use only cold-pressed olive, safflower, pumpkin, and canola oils for cooking and dressing foods. Never fry foods in oil or eat anything that is deep fried. Frying changes the chemical composition of food, making it highly carcinogenic.

Salt: Use sea salt in moderation as it contains essential trace minerals. Do not use regular table salt for cooking and seasoning.

Sugar: None. That is no typo! Do not use white or brown sugar or products with evaporated cane sugar and corn syrup. These simple carbs make your blood sugar levels spike up and drop down after 20 minutes, which means you feel fatigued and sluggish. Also avoid artificial sweeteners, which some studies have shown affect your ability to know when you have eaten enough. That is totally counterproductive!

Spices: Replace black pepper with red cayenne pepper, which has anti-inflammatory properties that help when you are trying to detoxify your body. You can also use curry, cumin, turmeric, and cinnamon.

Herbs: Cook with the freshest herbs you can find at the market. Freeze-dried products should be your second choice.

Condiments: Do not use prepared condiments such as ketchup, mustard, mayonnaise, salad dressings, etc.

Dressings: Try olive oil and lemon, with some fresh herbs and a little sea salt.

Drinks: Drink at least eight glasses of water a day. Ideally, you should drink half your body weight in ounces of water per day (body weight (in kg [lbs/2.2=kg] x 0.033 = how much water you should drink in liters). Use juice from half a fresh lemon for flavor. Do not drink soft drinks, sodas, sports drinks, coffee, decaf coffee, coffee substitutes, cocoa, alcohol, black teas, or green teas. All of them contain sugar, fake sugar, or caffeine. There is more about them in *Why Certain Foods Can Make You Fat* in chapter 4: *Improve Your Fat-itude*.

Herbal teas: All types are permitted: alfalfa, chamomile, cinnamon, clove, fennel, ginger, goldenseal, lemongrass, maitake, pau d'arco, peppermint, raspberry, or spearmint.

Continue Making Smart Choices

Bloating and weight gain can easily happen again if you do not pay close attention to your food intake the 3 days following the juicing. Besides the Flat Belly Tips given above, follow the menus listed below for the 3 days following the juicing when your intake should be between 1,200 and 1,300 calories.

Day Three

Upon rising:
1 glass water with fresh lemon
Peppermint tea
Breakfast:
1 cup plain yogurt with 1 tsp flaxseeds (ground)
Snack 1:
1 white grapefruit*
Lunch
Alpine Survival Salad (page 172)
Snack 2
1 white grapefruit*
Dinner
Stir-fried vegetables with grilled chicken (page 159)

Day Four

Upon rising:
1 glass water with fresh lemon
Peppermint tea
Breakfast
½ cup oatmeal made with brown rice milk and cinnamon
8 oz nonf. yogurt
2 tsp flaxseed (ground)
Snack 1
8 oz nonf. yogurt
6 almonds
Lunch
½ cup onions
2 small beets
1 ½ cups squash (summer)
2 cups broccoli
4 cups lettuce
1 egg
½ avocado
2 tsp Olive oil and lemon
Snack 2
1 egg
Dinner
20 med. spears asparagus
3 oz wild salmon
½ avocado

Day Five

Upon rising:
1 glass water with fresh lemon
Peppermint tea
Breakfast
1 cup carrot spread
1 slice rye bread
Snack 1
8 oz nonf. yogurt
1 tsp flaxseed (ground)
12 almonds
Lunch
½ cup sprouts
2 cups lettuce
1 cup tomatoes
1 cup peppers
2 cups kale
4 cups spinach
½ cup onion
½ avocado
1 tsp Olive oil and lemon
Snack 2
2 whole eggs
Dinner
6 oz chicken breast
2 cups yellow salad (page 171)
½ avocado
½ grapefruit*

* Check in with your doctor regarding consumption of grapefruits and your medication

After you completed the first 2 or 5 days of the *A Flat Belly – "Schnell" (fast)!* Program, go back to your *Choose Tomatoes Not Potatoes* (page 37) for *Alpine Eating with Fresh Air Foods* in chapter 3. How do you know if you want to do 2 days or 6 days? Use common sense. If you feel comfortable, continue the program. If you have difficulties with the sugar withdrawal go to the sample menu program on page 51.

Flat Belly Exercise Basics

Now that you have experienced the quick results of the flat belly anti-bloat plan, it is time to make the results permanent by making the right choices about long-term middle management: Choosing the right foods accounts for about 60% for your flat belly success. Activity and proper activation of the mid-section, or core, make up the rest of the equation. Daily activity massages your abdomen and therefore enhances the functioning of your digestive system.

4 Ways to Practice for a Flat Belly:

❶ All in to Be Thin

Activating your abdominal wall is as easy as pushing your belly button out and pulling it back in—and keeping it pulled in. If you just let your abdominals fall slack, you do not get the activation or tightening that creates stability for the spine. The result? An unstable environment for movement and a big-belly profile. When you pull your belly button in, you are tightening all the small muscles around your spine, which creates stability when you move; this stability can help prevent back issues.

Practice this flat belly exercise number 1 while sitting. Breathe out and pull the belly button in. Hold for 3 seconds. Breathe in and push the belly button out, followed by breathing out and pulling the belly button in. Repeat 10 times. If you master this sitting, try it standing on 1 leg to increase the challenge. This works the transverse abdominals or TVA and internal abdominal wall. If the TVA and internal abdominal wall becomes weak, it can no longer support the internal organs. If the abdominal wall can no longer provide support, the colon, liver, and stomach begin to drop, putting pressure on the rest of the digestive tract, uterus, and bladder. This can lead to increased menstrual pain, incontinence, and prostate-related problems. The medical term for this is Visceroptosis— a drop from the original, optimal position. A visible belly bulge might result.

❷ Doing the Abdominal Wall at the Office

Another way to practice TVA activation is to tie a leather string around your waist. A leather string is thicker, easy to tie a knot in, and does not stretch out like ordinary string can. Take that string and bring it around your waist. Pull in your belly button toward your spine as much as you can and hold it there. Tie a knot so that it feels comfortable while breathing. During your workout or for 1 hour during the day wear this string. Take it off after 60 minutes. Look at your belly, and you will see 1 of 2 things—you have a bright red mark from the string or just a very light imprint from the string. The first option tells you that you need to work on your mid-body activation and maintaining it. If this is the case, you can start immediately. Remind yourself when you sit, stand, walk, or bend over to pull your belly button in. No crunches required!

❹ Practice Your Kegels

As I explained in an earlier chapter, Kegel exercises are not just squeezing your butt together or pulling your stomach in, nor are they about pushing out and thrusting out your lower abdomen. The Kegel exercises activate the pelvic girdle through an inward and up movement. This is not just for women! Guys, it is just as important for you, especially if you lift heavy weights.

You can find the deeper internal activations by using the muscles you use to stop the flow of urine. Be careful because you do not want to start actually retaining urine; it is just a way to help you identify the right muscles. You want to be able to hold the activation for 10 seconds, but you may have to work up to that. Try holding them 6 times a day.

Do the Kegels anywhere, even while you are waiting on line at the supermarket. No one will ever know, but you will be doing a world of good for your mid-body.

❺ Balance with Your Belly

Start on your hands and knees on the floor; make sure to align your hands directly under your shoulders. Simultaneously extend the right arm in front of you and the left leg behind you, forming an even horizontal line. The more you activate your abdominal wall and pelvic floor, the easier it will be to balance. Lower back to starting position and repeat with your left arm and right leg. Repeat 10 times for a balanced core, mid-body, and a flatter stomach.

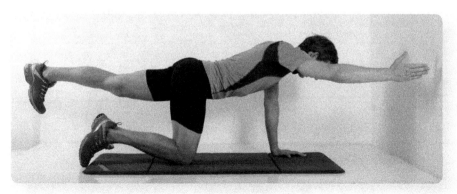

ALPINE
WEIGHT LOSS
SECRETS

Worksheet 10

The right foods are key to flattening your belly. Instead of eating foods that could possibly make you bloated (lack of enzymes) or constipated (lack of fiber), eat an improved version. Rolled or steel-cut oats instead of white toast for breakfast. A grilled chicken breast instead of packaged seasoned sausages. Fresh bananas instead of tiramisu. You get the idea. What are your better belly foods?

Current flat belly damaging foods:

....

....

....

....

....

....

Flat belly improving foods:

....

....

....

....

....

....

ALPINE
WEIGHT LOSS
SECRETS

Worksheet 11

Multi-task your belly exercises. Upon rising I pull in my stomach and push it out again for 15 repetitions. Or every time I take the stairs, I activate my pelvic floor to practice the Kegels. Schedule your own times to multi-task and work these muscles.

Places of pelvic floor activation:

....

....

....

....

....

....

Places of abdominal activation:

....

....

....

....

....

....

1
2
3
4
5
6
7
8
9
10
11

Worksheet 12

Think back into your past. When was the last time you really wanted to accomplish a goal? What did you do to achieve this? How did you organize yourself? Write down below what you did to accomplish your goal and apply your same skill set to the 2-Day Alpine Cleansing Cure.

Past achieved goal:

....

....

....

....

....

....

How did you achieve it? (Write down managerial and organizational skills.)

....

....

....

....

....

....

ALPINE
WEIGHT LOSS
SECRETS

7 Best Flat Belly Boosters

What are you waiting for? These 7 tips can help you boost your flat belly schnell today:

❶ **Drink citrus.** Lemon in water is a liver cleanser, fat emulsifier, and high in B vitamins (important in energy conversion on a cellular level) if you include some white of the peel.

❷ **Walk thin.** Sit thin and exercise thin. What do I mean by that? Practice the Kegels while walking or sitting. Activate the abdominal wall while standing in line, while waiting at a stop light, as you climb the stairs.

❸ **Do not chew gum.** It promotes swallowing air, which can bloat your belly.

❹ **Drink (water) before you eat.** Or order a broth-based soup before your main course. Studies have shown that hot liquid before main courses gives you a faster sense of satisfaction. In short, fewer calories will be consumed.

❺ **Buy a waist string today.** Tie it around your waist so you can see how often you let your abdominal muscles go slack. Use the string for 1 hour tomorrow.

❻ **Start the Flat Belly Tips.** Guaranteed: you feel and will see a difference after 4 days.

❼ **Ramp it up.** Try 7 days without fruit sugars. Only lemons, limes, or grapefruit*. Why? Yeast is evil, and yeast is fed by sugar and alcohol.

* Check in with your doctor if you take medication regarding the consumption of grapefruit.

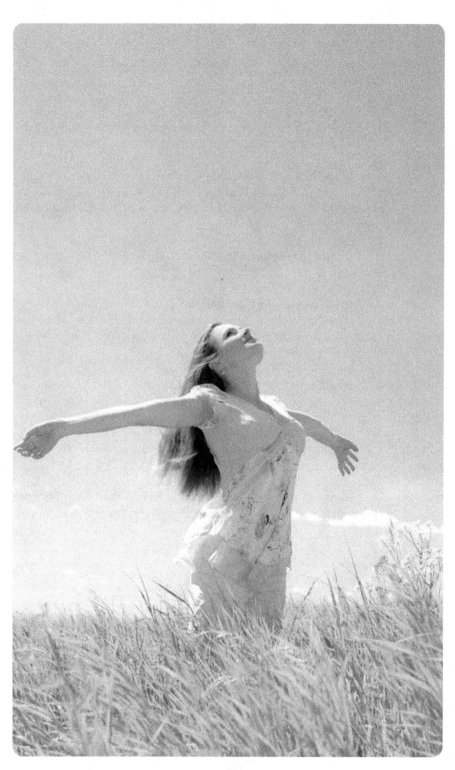

ALPINE
WEIGHT LOSS
SECRETS

Chapter 9

THE JOY OF LIVING: THINK AND GROW THIN

1
2
3
4
5
6
7
8
9
10
11

This program is not just about food and exercise. However, a healthy by-product of the focus on your fitness level and the quality of your nutrition is that it helps clear your mind of mental stress and promotes clarity.

Steve Jobs once said something that changed my life. "You can't connect the dots looking forward," he said in a commencement address. "You can only connect them looking backwards, so you have to trust that the dots will some-how connect in your future. You have to trust in something—your gut, destiny, life, karma, or whatever—because believing that the dots will connect down the road will give you the confidence to follow your heart, even when it leads you off the well-worn path, and that will make all the difference."

His words made me analyze my life's direction. I listed all my accomplishments, jobs, and hobbies. The ones that excited me and made me happiest had to do with helping people to change to look and feel better. With my degree in finance, I was working on Wall Street, but at that moment, I knew that wasn't the right place for me.

My next step was to quit and incorporate my own business. You might find yourself in a situation that you don't like. Add a few years of stress, depression, and unhappiness, which can be a by-product of your daily struggles, and you will need to find other outlets for happiness. This might be escapism such as constantly reading in your free time (romantic books) or watching videos and movies, which are activities that are not active. Then add mental exhaustion from keeping up with your work, your children, and your relationship. Reach for chocolate, ice cream, cookies, chips, or cupcakes is an attempt to keep your energy up and to drown the emotional unhappiness that is stuck in the throat. Many have placed themselves in this kind situation and will need much more than exercise and nutritional changes to get back on track.

ALPINE
WEIGHT LOSS
SECRETS

7 Questions to Consider

The fresh air, the activity, and their community all contribute to Alpine people's feeling of comfort. Alpine people are happy people. Ever been to Sedona? Boulder? Aspen? Those are other Alpine places where people are happy. You will get the time of the day if you are lost, have a question answered, or just have a friendly chat. How can you get to this state of happiness?

Here are your seven questions that can help you focus on taking care of your wants and needs again and moving in the direction where you should be:

Question 1: What is it that I am supposed to do with my life?

Whatever it is, it is never too late. To find out what you are really supposed to do with your life, you need to tune out all the external voices around you such as TV, radio, news, magazines, and anything else out there. The best exercise would be to lock yourself into a dark room (bathrooms work best) where no light or sound can stimulate you and listen to your thoughts. Lie on your back with closed or covered eyes, earplugs in your ears, and let your thoughts wander around this question. Let it come to you. Have a pen and paper ready to jot things down in the dark. If you fall asleep, that is okay because you need the rest. Repeat this until you have your answer.

For me, the moment of realization came when I noted all my past decisions (hairdresser, culinary arts degree, fitness and nutrition certifications, and a master's in nutrition) and realized that I need to (have to) help other people. My time spent in an office helping 1 person make money was not it. I gave notice the next day, and my focus became helping other people to feel, look, and be younger naturally. The dark room exercise revealed to me that helping other people is my obligation.

Find it strange to sit in a quiet dark room? Thomas Edison, the inventor of the light bulb, used this method to look for solutions when attempts failed. He never gave up. We can thank him for light bulbs.

Question 2: Am I in the right place at this moment?

For whatever reason, we end up in the wrong places. This can be a physical place, a position at a job, or a destination that we thought would be right. Sometimes we end up in places because we gave up following our purpose in life to pursue the life we were really meant to lead. In my situation it was Austria and my destination was the United States. For another client, it was not to operate a trading desk but to be a trader. Another client, a doctor, knew that her calling was as a musician. For an editor, it was the place to become a doctor. For an actress, it was to be an opera singer. Ask yourself that question and give yourself the right answer. Be honest when you answer this question. Allow yourself to give yourself the right answer! Let it come out and don't ignore it.

ALPINE
WEIGHT LOSS
SECRETS

Question 3: What makes me happy?

Integrity might be the most important value that contributes to your happiness. Integrity is not a value in itself but rather the value that guarantees that other values are real values. Once you grasp your integrity it will be easier to follow your commitments to follow your goals. And the higher your integrity, the stronger the feeling of satisfaction you will experience with everything you do.

Decide that you want to be a respected man or woman. Crystallize your values in each area in your life and stick with them. Live up to them and don't lower your bar. Again, raise your standards. To help you to clarify your values, make a list of values that you really believe in and stand for. Then analyze the actions that would make you follow those values and the actions that move you away from those values. Integrity and happiness come by following your values and not moving away from them. It is your personal prayer, mission statement, or law to live by.

Question 4: What is it that I really want to do?

This is probably a question that is answered differently by the generation born before 1964 and the upcoming generation. Mothers' or fathers' footsteps do not have to be followed anymore. Yet there was a time where parents demanded children follow in their footsteps. Some among us do live a life that is not ours but was created by somebody else. This might be lawyers who wanted to be doctors or doctors who wanted to be entrepreneurs. Farmers who wanted a city job might be another example. What is it that you really want to do? Take a trip? Change your profession? Take some time off? Find a way to do it. Don't procrastinate because you never know if tomorrow might be too late.

Question 5: Am I happy with the direction in which I am going with my life?

Check in daily. Ask yourself this question in the morning. There might be days when you are happy and other days where you are not. If there are more days when you are not, go deeper. What is it that bothers you? How can you improve it right now? To be happy and in control with the direction of your life you need to check in with your emotions. Your emotions are anything but joyful when you are in the process of weight loss. In fact, you're depressed and perhaps angry and disappointed.

How long does it take to change your emotions? If you change the meaning you give something, you can immediately change your emotions. Internal communication and the right questions can change your emotions instantly and, with them, your focus. The most powerful way to change the meaning you give something, say, weight loss, is to change your focus. And since focus is controlled by questions that you ask yourself, the key is to ask yourself quality questions. It is simple: just ask a different question, and you change your focus. For instance, instead of asking why you can't lose weight, which may make you even more depressed, you could ask how you could appreciate your good health and better serve your body to stay young and healthy at this moment. This question will lead immediately to a positive emotion (no guilt, no despair) and will encourage you to adopt strategies that are helpful to you.

Asking the right question can be your solution to changing your immediate strategies. Even better, this approach will result in continuing improvements that will help you find the direction to take in your life.

Question 6: What will my future be?

The present does not determine your future. Your future needs planning. Time management is the key to success. Manage your time on a daily, weekly, monthly, and yearly schedule. Build lists that you follow. Nothing is perfect the first time you create it on paper. Keep revising and improving it. Plan the steps that are necessary to get you there. And revise them again if you find a better way. It is fluid intelligence. Things do change around you, and you need to adapt. This applies to your work environment, technology, and your relationships with your partner and children too. Life changes, and you must adapt. Stay flexible.

Question 7: What have I done today that contributes to my better future?

When you have your goals for where you want to be in the future this will be your first step. You must move toward this goal. It takes action. Without action nothing will be moving in your chosen direction. If you expect otherwise, that would be called insanity (expecting a different outcome while doing the same thing over and over again). Everyday, before you go to bed, answer this question with at least 3 things you have done to create a better future. If you have less than 3, you better ramp up your implementation and get it done. And this can refer not just to your physical goals but also to your financial or relation-ship goals.

If you don't know where you are going with your life, you may wake up one day and find yourself somewhere (or someone) that you don't want to be. In my experience, this is when people feel stressed and use food as an outlet. It snowballs. Suddenly they feel too tired to exercise.

Ask yourself these 7 questions and analyze your answers! See if you're on track. Stress causes oxidative damage on your cells that ages you. It is time to limit emotional stress to reduce cellular stress! Take control! Once again, change your mind, change your body, AND your life.

Worksheet 13

Have you done something today? What is nagging you? Is there something that you'd like to change but feel you can't and therefore you eat, turn on the TV, or escape into books? Come, stay with me. Just turn off the stimuli and listen to yourself again. Listen to your body and your thoughts. Let them talk. Right now, write down 3 areas you want to work on. You can do it. Do it now:

What is coming as the first thing (focus) in your mind that you want to change?

Focus of interest 1:

....

....

....

....

Focus of interest 2:

....

....

....

....

Focus of interest 3:

....

....

....

....

1
2
3
4
5
6
7
8
9
10
11

Now, write down what your goal is in the areas of focus of interest that you have chosen:

Goal for interest 1:

....

....

....

....

....

....

Goal for interest 2:

....

....

....

....

....

....

Goal for interest 3:

....

....

....

....

....

....

ALPINE
WEIGHT LOSS
SECRETS

Now that you have thought about your goals, the next step requires a little bit more thought. Write down 20 action steps for each goal that you'd like to accomplish. Yes, push your buttons. Do NOT stop before you have 20 solid steps for each single goal. Think hard.

	Goal 1	Goal 2	Goal 3
Action step 1:			
Action step 2:			
Action step 3:			
Action step 4:			
Action step 5:			
Action step 6:			
Action step 7:			
Action step 8:			
Action step 9:			
Action step 10:			
Action step 11:			
Action step 12:			
Action step 13:			
Action step 14:			
Action step 15:			
Action step 16:			
Action step 17:			
Action step 18:			
Action step 19:			
Action step 20:			

What you just created is a road map that you can follow. Implement the steps that you have just created. These are your solutions to overcoming your obstacles. Come back after 2 weeks and see what you have implemented. If you find it was difficult to implement the steps, adjust them. Keep in mind this is a flexible process. But start creating momentum toward your goal objectives. "Most people in life don't have a goal and aim around the target and end up nowhere," remarked Brian Tracey in his book *Goals*, and I fully agree. Pick up his book to become more inspired.

8 Attitude Adjusters: How to Make a Bad Day Good

There are times when the going gets rough. There are good days and bad days. I tell my clients who have a bad day to think of bad days as a big black hole that will suck you in. On the bottom is a huge trampoline. The deeper the hole, the higher you will bounce back. And there are many holes and trampolines that you will fall into during your life. All of them will bounce you back again.

Here are attitude adjusters that can help you to make a bad day good:

❶　　　**Exercise. A given. Just move.** Do something for yourself and be active to get the endorphins going. This can be doing push-ups, walking stairs, going to the gym or for a walk. A client of mine said once that when she has a lot of issues going on she goes for a longer walk but doesn't run. Walking helps her to clear her mind but running does not have the same effect. While walking you can focus on your thoughts, place the issues on the side, enjoy the environment around you, and focus on your breathing. With each 4 steps you can train your confidence by chanting I AM POWERFUL or I AM STRONG. Inhale during the first steps and exhale during the next 4 steps.

❷　　　**Be nice to someone.** Instant gratification can be accomplished by picking up the phone and saying something nice to someone. Do not send an e-mail. You need to hear the other person's response. Even better would be to say it in person. The first rule of making yourself happy is to make other people happy. A nice response from another person will calm you and help you to focus on positive areas in your life again.

❸　　　**Stop beating yourself up.** Ever had someone go on and on about her or his issues and you feel enough already? Your advice might have been to simply say, "Just move on." Moving on is sometimes hard, but it works. Think about the positives in your life or the positive actions that you have done this day, and continue with your positive thoughts and take actions accordingly.

ALPINE
WEIGHT LOSS
SECRETS

❹ **Snap out of it.** It might have been eating obsessively or being on a path of bad luck. Both of which can lead you to reach for food for comfort. Change your thinking. Do something unexpected. Just change the path of your thinking. For example, stop your compulsive eating and invite your friends to cook a new raw food recipe. Switch from processed food to raw foods. Another simple strategy is to think of your role model and ask yourself: What would person X do?

❺ **Take a power nap.** Taking a nap rejuvenates your systems and your body. It is as if you're starting your second day. It helps you to see an upsetting situation in a new light. It might still upset you but much less than it did before.

❻ **Laugh.** In a time where we have so much access to infor-mation you can pick and choose. Sad? Screwed up? Depressed? Beating yourself up? Go to youtube.com and look for the comedy section. Find the best rated videos and watch for 15 minutes. Time yourself. It is really fun and addicting at the same time. Your mood will change instantly.

❼ **Change your point of view.** You can learn from every situation. You can learn from a good day as well as from a bad day. You alone determine whether something is good or bad. Try to find a learning situ-ation in a day gone insane. That is a skill to develop and will come in handy to see the good in things. No matter how bad it might be.

❽ **Edit your vocabulary.** Bad can have many different meanings, for example, challenging, interesting, or eventful. Communicate with yourself in a new way. Avoid the word bad and call it interesting or any other word you might choose. The word interesting gives you much more room to explore and discover the real meaning of your day or your situation.

My advice to you is to relax. Yes, take it easy. During recessions or burst economic bubbles, stress increases and challenging situations arrive. And with them come strokes, heart attacks, and a rise in blood pressure. Yes, all 3 can be prevented through regular exercise and proper nutrition.

Stress management is another very important factor in your health. Stop and smell the roses. Take it easier and enjoy the moments life presents you. Always ask what you can learn from this situation.

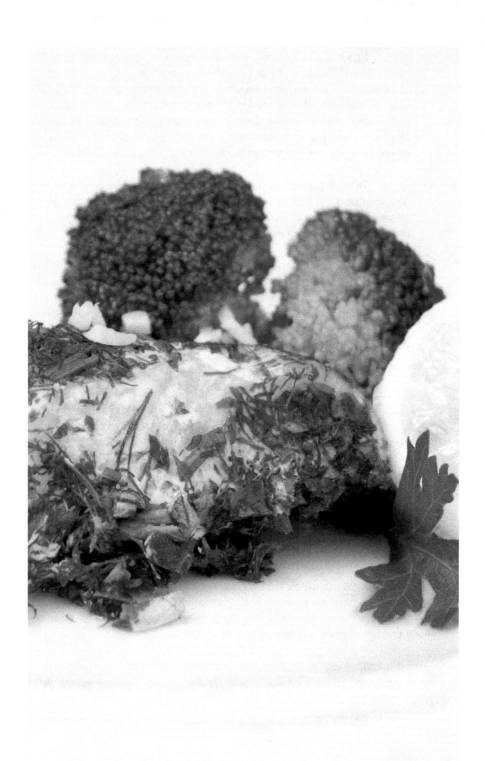

ALPINE
WEIGHT LOSS
SECRETS

Chapter 10

"HUDRY WUSCH:" EAT YOURSELF THIN

By now you know that Fresh Air Foods that are unprocessed, plant based, and possibly organic will not only trim pounds, they will brighten your mood, jump-start your energy, and turn back your aging clock. Okay, fine, but how do you transform such fresh air ingredients into tasty meals? Two words: *Hudry Wusch*. (That means easy and simple as 1, 2, and 3). Even if you're not a cook, you can make these delicious recipes. It takes just 3 to 4 items to make a delicious meal, which makes shopping easier, drastically reduces preparation time, and saves money too. In fact, it's faster to cook or assemble your dinner than order takeout. This chapter contains 60 of my most popular recipes so that you can eat yourself thin.

Explore and discover. Diet is always associated with starvation and restriction. Not here. You must eat to feed your cells on a cellular level. When you eat food that is not as close as possible to the earth and air, you will still be hungry and looking for more food after a few hours. This program is designed to feed your cells on a cellular level. It might happen that you eat more the first days of the program. Yet when you start feeding your cells, your body will adjust to a natural calorie requirement that will be the right amount for you and your lifestyle. Don't drop below 1,200 calories (women) and 1,800 calories (men) for weight loss with an active activity schedule.

Clients ask me if they should stick rigorously to those calorie loads even when they are not hungry and just consuming 1,000 calories when they have excessive fat tissue stored. Should they force themselves to eat those additional calories or not? As a simple rule, if you maintain your blood sugar levels with 3 meals and 2 snacks, you don't have to, as long you don't start rampaging the following day or in the evening. Stored fat tissue is energy that can be accessed. By eating the foods that are beneficial for your body to maintain an efficient metabolism (enzymes are the key here), your body will adjust to it by eating less and accessing the stored fat. This is what you want. My experience has shown that when this happens, individuals who eat a fewer calories for several days will eat a little bit more for the next day or 2.

This is called the zigzag approach and is a natural occurrence. Just learn to listen to your body. Eat when you are hungry. Stop when you have had enough. Don't eat when you are not. This program will help you to get back in touch with your natural calorie adjustments without counting calories. I highly recommend that you don't count calories during the first 14 days. Then, when you feel you need a structured program, go to the sample menu on page 51 and follow it.

None of the recipes give you a calorie count. It is not necessary when you go through the first 14 days. Rather it is necessary to follow the program as given. Cheating will not help you accomplish your goal. All the information that is provided will help you to accomplish the program with ease. I know you can do it just as many others in your situation have. Just relax. It will happen. Stay focused and on target.

A Fast New Way to Cook: 60 Simple, Delicious Recipes for Breakfast, Snacks, Lunch, Dinner and Desserts

The best part about these Look, Learn, Do recipes is that each of them is correlated to the Alpine Eating Plan. The Look, Learn, Do recipes are very flavorful and all the food items are interchangeable. You don't want to eat the same thing over and over again, and these recipes will give you flexibility. It is important to rotate your foods just as you do your exercise program.

It can be difficult to cook every day, but these recipes and suggested foods are also easy to prepare and enjoyable to eat. Trust me, you can do it for 14 days or find delis or restaurants that follow your guidelines.

As soon as you learn some of the basics in these recipes (they are even funny as well...you'll see!), you will be able to become more creative in your approach. Remember to try different things and explore new tastes! Who cares if you screw up? That can happen. So be it.

BREAKFAST

You have heard it over and over again: BREAKFAST IS THE MOST IMPORTANT MEAL OF YOUR DAY. It's a meal that should contain protein, carbohydrates, and fats, but that doesn't mean you have to eat them all at the same time. Try lingering over breakfast. You can start out with oatmeal, and 2 hours later have some hard-boiled eggs. Break it up if you need to, but most importantly, pay attention to your digestion as you eat. Certain food combinations simply do not belong together or just may not agree with you. Again, if you need a structured program, use the sample menu on page 51.

Keep an open mind. Don't even think about telling me you don't like anything on this list until you have at least given these suggestions a try. If you truly cannot stomach any of my delicious breakfast recipes, there is only one thing to do: eat your dinner in the morning. That's right, you heard me. There is nothing wrong with eating salad, arugula, spinach, or other greens with fish, chicken, or turkey in the morning. There are actually many benefits to eating this way. For example, you immediately give your digestive enzymes a jump-start for the day.

BREAKFAST OPTIONS

WHOLE GRAIN BREADS
Who said you can't eat bread? There are so many delicious varieties to choose from—rye, spelt, brown rice, or kamut—and they are sugar and yeast free. When I arrived in the States in 1997, it was difficult to find anything but white bread. Fortunately that's not true today. White bread is a big fluff compared to the sturdy and dense bread we eat back home. Take 2 slices in the morning, toast them, and smear with hummus. It's so comforting to eat warm, whole grain bread in the morning with a little something on top. You're getting protein, essential fiber, minerals, and even beneficial fats from the hummus and carbohydrates in the grains. When you shop, read the label of ingredients in the bread.

EGGS
Nothing is simpler than eggs in the morning. How many variations do you know? Whether they are scrambled, poached, or hard boiled, find the kind you love best and enjoy a great protein boost in the morning. Some people have trouble digesting eggs. So if you're one of those people, cook them the way that works for you. Most people can handle hard-boiled eggs with no problem, and they are great to have handy for a quick snack.

TIP! Beware of the bedeviling deli eggs! Have you ever considered what they are cooked in? Probably vegetable oil, lard, butter, or bacon fat. No wonder many individuals can't digest them and feel bloated afterwards! When possible, try to make and enjoy your eggs at home for the healthiest option as many delis and diners use hydrogenated vegetable oils!

FRUITS
As mentioned earlier, you can add fruit after the first 14 days of the Alpine Eating Plan. Go for local and seasonal fruits, in addition to lemons, limes, and grapefruit that are available all year. Have seasonal fruit with yogurt and some ground flaxseeds to provide you protein, fats, and carbohydrates.

BREAKFAST RECIPES

MISH-MASH OMELET

Ingredients:
3 eggs
1 bunch sautéed fresh spinach
Extra virgin olive oil
Sea salt (always use sparingly)

Beat the eggs with a fork until liquid. If you like, add a little brown rice milk to make the omelet fluffier.

Sauté the prewashed spinach in a heated skillet sprinkled with olive oil. After placing the spinach in the skillet, cover it until the spinach is wilted, and remove to a separate plate. Rinse the skillet briefly with cold water, add a spritz of olive oil again, and reheat.

Stir-fry the beaten eggs by pouring them into the heated skillet and allow to sit without stirring for 2 minutes. Then place the sautéed spinach on top. Remove from range and place in a 450°F oven for about 7 to 10 minutes. You will know the omelet is finished when the liquid on top has evaporated. Consider making a double portion because it's even more delicious the next day or serve it as an egg pizza dinner the following evening. To serve, slice like a pizza.

TIP! Change things around by varying the vegetables you use. Try broccoli, asparagus, or whatever tickles your fancy but still satisfies your daily nutritional needs.

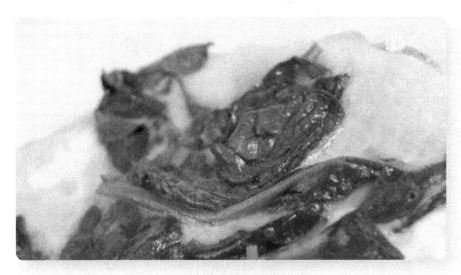

HEIDI'S SECRET

Let me introduce a breakfast drink for anyone who absolutely does not have time for breakfast. Trust me, you have time for this. I have heard clients say, "Stefan, I still want space for the foods I love in the morning. But this gets rid of my hunger. I don't have room for more." Well, that isn't a bad thing.

Ingredients:
2 parts of organic nonfat or low-fat yogurt
1 part water or rice milk
2 tsp organic almond butter
¼ tsp ground cinnamon
¼ tsp ground turmeric

Blend two parts yogurt and one part water, soymilk, or rice milk in a blender.
Season the blend with almond butter, ground cinnamon, and ground turmeric to taste. (I'll leave the measurements up to you!)
Serve, drink, and enjoy after blending for another 30 seconds.

TIP! Add some cayenne pepper and enjoy after lunch as a digestive aid. Heidi's Secret also makes a great midmorning or afternoon snack. If you are not on the 14 days of the Alpine Eating Plan, add some local fruits.

THE SOUND OF YOGURT

The power of yogurt is even mentioned in the movie Star Wars, so just think what it can do for your digestion. The friendly bacteria in yogurt aid your digestion, leaving your body with more energy to speed up your metabolism.

Ingredients:
1½ cups organic nonfat or low-fat yogurt
2 tablespoons organic raw almond butter
¼ tsp ground cinnamon

Place the yogurt in the center of your nicest bowl, the one you like to eat out of most.
Pour 2 tablespoons almond butter over it. Make a nice pattern with the almond butter, and add some cinnamon for decoration.
Serve... oops! It's gone already.

TIP! Stir yogurt and almond butter together so that it looks like hazelnut ice cream. Or, instead of almond butter, use almond halves or walnuts.

OATMEAL

So delicious. Remember the replacement theory? Trick yourself into how good everything tastes, and soon it will taste good.

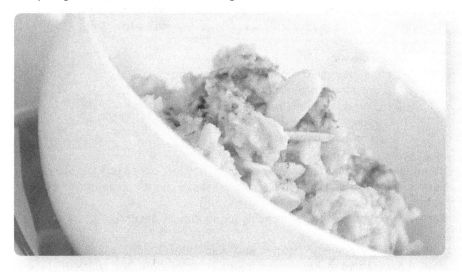

Ingredients:
2 cups rolled oats
3 cups rice milk
¼ tsp ground cinnamon

Soak the oatmeal in rice milk overnight in a covered pot or container.
Heat up the soaked oatmeal in the morning for about 3 minutes and add the ground cinnamon. If it is too dry, add more liquid. Try it one time to see if you like it not cooked. A hint! Uncooked oatmeal with raisins, apples, and fresh lemon juice is the famous Bircher Muesli from Austria.
Serve your oatmeal in your favorite bowl. Hudry Wusch, and enjoy.

TIP! Use the leftover oatmeal from the day before and add some of The Sound of Yogurt. Also, start exploring other grains or mix them in with your oatmeal. And no, instant oatmeal doesn't count. When you read the ingredients you won't believe what is inside.

SNACKS

How can you make the program work on the run or on the fly?
Here are some ideas:

- **Nuts** – easy to eat and to carry, and constantly accessible. For nuts ideas look at Category 1 under Proteins to get ideas. Of course, don't eat them if you are allergic to nuts.

- **Plain yogurt** – easy to find.

- **Green, red, or orange peppers** – you just need to plan ahead to have them ready for you. Cut them in slices and enjoy.

- **White grapefruit** – Don't get your sports bag or handbag dirty. They come in their own bag, and it's called the peel.

- **Vegetable juices** – easy to buy almost anywhere. Always buy freshly squeezed only, not from concentrate.

- **Hard-boiled eggs** – so easy to do yourself, and many delis and markets now sell them too.

- **Yams** – cut them into small pieces and roast them with a little bit of cinnamon on top; they will make your taste buds jump! Take them with you in a little bag when you are on the run.

TIP! Have a look at www.happycow.net. This site lists restaurants and shopping possibilities for food to eat on the run that are available on the Alpine Eating Plan. Also, you can search online for health-food stores or health-food restaurants to find those in your area. There are many solutions that exist, and they are for YOU to discover.

LOOK, LEARN, DO RECIPES:

LUNCH, DINNER, AND DESSERTS

These recipes use all the ingredients that are essential to successfully complete the 14 days of the Alpine Eating Plan without sugars, including fruit sugars. Most important, these recipes are meant to be healthful, quick, and delicious. *Hudry Wusch!* That is the best part.

ORGANIC CHICKEN with
BUTTERNUT SQUASH IN A GINGER CURRY SAUCE

Look

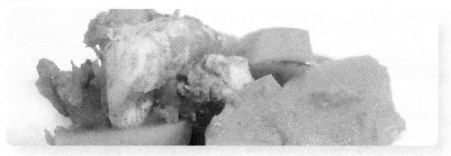

Learn

Ingredients:

1 organic chicken breast
1 medium butternut squash
2 tablespoons Indian curry
1 medium piece fresh ginger root
Extra virgin olive oil
Sea salt

Benefits:

This meal requires nothing more than chopping. In less than 4 minutes, you should be able to chop all of the ingredients and then let simmer while you play with your daughter, son, dog, or maybe just put your feet up and relax. Have you experienced the Mountain Program already? Well, then, you'll be happy to know squash helps relieve pain. But besides pain relief, squash reduces inflammation and soothes the stomach. Summer squash is lower in calories than winter squash, which is higher in carbohydrates.

Do

Hudry Wusch Technique:

Chop the squash and chicken into equal pieces.
Sauté chicken in olive oil in a hot pan for about 2 minutes. Turn after one minute. Add the squash, curry, ginger, and sea salt, and cover.
Cook for another 2 minutes, and then add 2 cups of water to the pan. Cook for another 3 minutes, and then lower the flame and let simmer until the squash gets soft and the water turns into its own ginger curry sauce. Call and invite me over when you make this dish. In a flash you will have a new dinner guest.

HERBED WILD SALMON FILLET with
FARM-FRESH BROCCOLI and SHORT-GRAIN BROWN RICE

Look

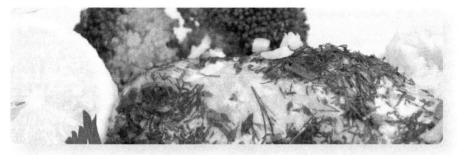

Learn

Ingredients:

1 wild salmon fillet
1 broccoli crown, broken into florets
2 cups brown rice
1 lemon, freshly squeezed
2 chopped garlic cloves
Fresh dill, sage, and parsley, finely chopped
Extra virgin olive oil
Sea salt

Benefits:

Brainpower take notice: The natural fats in this meal increase brain function, reduce the severity of migraine headaches, and, most importantly, reduce joint inflammation from arthritis. The herbs used in this recipe are known to ease sore throats and indigestion; they also help increase circulation and lower blood pressure. The bottom line: this meal is great for losing weight and gives you more brainpower. It's the perfect meal for a body that sits all day.

Do

Hudry Wusch Technique:

Cook 1 part rice to 2 parts water in a rice cooker or pot. Add sea salt and olive oil. If you use a pot, bring the rice and water to a boil, then turn down and allow to simmer. Cooking time: approximately 15 minutes. If you are using a rice cooker, let it cook until it turns itself off.
Blanch the broccoli florets by bringing water to a boil, and add the broccoli florets. After no more than 2 minutes remove them from the pot and drain.

1
2
3
4
5
6
7
8
9
10
11

Splash olive oil, lemon juice, sea salt, and garlic on the steaming broccoli. Bake the fish after preparing it the following way: Place the washed salmon fillet in the middle of a piece of parchment paper and cover with the chopped herbs. Fold the parchment paper tightly so the fish and the herbs are fully enclosed and can cook in their own juice. Place them in the preheated 450°F oven for approximately 15 to 20 minutes. Serve all together on 1 plate.

TIP! Afraid to smell like garlic? Don't worry about it. The fresh lemon juice will counteract the garlic. Chewing parsley helps as well. And what's more important: your health, your weight loss, and your energy or a little hint of garlic?

SAUTEED CHICKEN with
FARM-FRESH KALE and a SLICE of RYE BREAD

Look

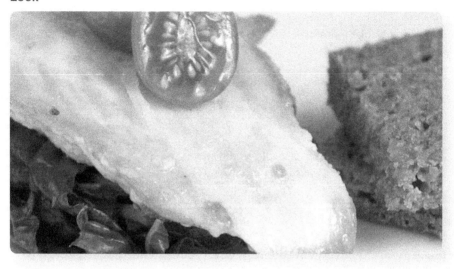

Learn

Ingredients:
1 cage-free boneless chicken breast
1 bunch organic kale
1 slice yeast-free, sugar-free rye bread
Extra virgin olive oil
Sea salt

Benefits:
This meal takes no time at all! In less than 7 minutes, you will be ready to dig into a nutritious meal that contains amino acids to help you grow and maintain lean muscles while you continue to exercise. The minerals and vitamins contained in kale and rye provide an excellent defense against stress, and fiber helps fight off blisters and bone loss disorders. Huh? Yes, the easily assimilated calcium, the lysine, and B vitamins in kale fight stress and sores. The bottom line: this meal is great for people with no time, further reducing the stress and worry over what to eat. It cooks up fast and provides the right nutrition to keep your insulin levels up.

Do

Hudry Wusch Technique:
Sauté the seasoned chicken in a hot pan for approximately 2 minutes on each

side, until it is golden brown. Remove chicken, add water to the remaining bits to deglaze your pan, and create a delicious sauce. Heat for 30 seconds.

Steam sauté the dripping wet kale by placing it in a hot pan after cutting it into thick strips. Cover and let the evaporating heat steam the kale. Turn the kale after 1 minute, and let it cook another 2 minutes. Turn the burner off, season with salt, and let it sit another 1 to 2 minutes.

Serve the chicken, the kale, and the bread on a big plate. Then relax and think back on all the good things that have happened to you today.

TIP! If you don't like kale, substitute one item of the vegetable bonanza starting on page 167. Hey, you can change the grain to your liking as well.

ORGANIC WHITE GROUND TURKEY BURGER with ORGANIC BROCCOLI

Look

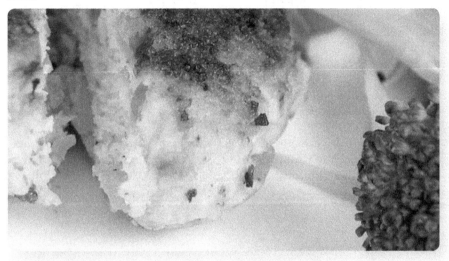

Learn

Ingredients:

2 lbs ground white organic turkey

1 onion

2 carrots

1 broccoli crown, broken into florets

1 lemon, fresh-squeezed juice

1 slice rye bread

Extra virgin olive oil

Sea salt

Benefits:

Turkey and chicken contain only 11% fat with the skin, and only 4% to 5% without the skin, while beef contains up to 30% and 40% fat. Hey, it would not be an issue about the fat if it was unsaturated, but as we know, the drama is about the saturated fats (animal fats). Still, turkey or chicken is a far better choice than beef for weight loss. Besides that, turkey (like eggs) contains amino acids, zinc, iron, potassium, phosphorus, and some of the B vitamins. Oh, yes, don't forget all the antioxidants in the onion, carrots, and broccoli, which help make your immune and cardiovascular systems function at 100%. Remember, you are building a body to take you into your 60s, 70s, 80s, and hopefully beyond, so you had better start preparing now!

Do

Hudry Wusch Technique:

Dice the carrots and onions. Mix them with the turkey and season with sea salt. Then form equal, hand-sized burgers. TIP! Use an ice-cream scoop for portion sizes. Cook the burgers by placing them into a hot pan covered slightly with olive oil. Cook until well done.

Blanch the broccoli florets; do this by cutting the crown into smaller pieces and placing them into boiling water for no more than 2 minutes; remove and drain. Splash olive oil, lemon juice, sea salt, and garlic on the steaming broccoli.

Slice the rye bread and place it on a serving plate with the broccoli and turkey burger. Voila! A delicious meal in 20 minutes or less!

TIP! The burgers are great to travel with during the week, if you think about bringing your lunch to work, or if you are on a heavy work schedule. This is much better tasting than any takeout, and you know what is inside.

ROAST CHICKEN with
FRESH ITALIAN VEGTABLE STUFFING

Look

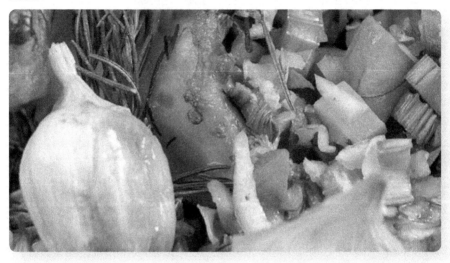

Learn

Ingredients:
1 cage-free whole chicken
5 cups diced carrots
5 cups diced celery
1 diced red onion
1 bunch fresh rosemary
Extra virgin olive oil
Sea salt

Benefits:
Chicken contains all the eight amino acids that help you grow lean muscle tissue, but of course it won't happen without exercise, as mentioned earlier. The carrot, celery, and onion are high in antioxidants and are delicious when roasted in the chicken. Additionally, celery is well known for weight loss and en-hances sex drive. So careful with the celery—it's more powerful than you think!

Do

Hudry Wusch Technique:
Dice all the vegetables and mix in a bowl. Season the mixture with olive oil and sea salt.

Stuff the washed chicken (that has been dried with a paper towel and rubbed with olive oil and sea salt) with the prepared diced vegetable mixture. Place the chicken in a baking pan and stick the sprigs of rosemary under the wings, inside the vegetable stuffing, and underneath the chicken.

Roast the chicken at 450°F until the skin is golden brown, for approximately 45 minutes. Slice the chicken and serve it with the stuffing and rosemary. The leftovers are great to nibble on during the week and perfect to take to work for lunch.

TIP! Try placing several whole, unpeeled garlic cloves in the pan around the chicken while roasting. Once golden brown, they will be hot and soft and can be mashed into a flavorful, healthy spread.

QUINOA SALAD with
ORGANIC FARM-FRESH VEGTABLES

Look

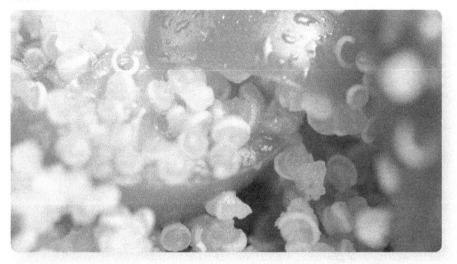

Learn

Ingredients:

3 cups quinoa

1 red onion, cut lengthwise

1 broccoli crown, prepared into florets

1 bunch organic spinach

1 small tomato

1 lemon, fresh-squeezed juice

1 small glass jar of anchovies, cut into small pieces

Extra virgin olive oil

Benefits:

All whole grains are complex carbohydrates that promote energy and maintain insulin levels. Additionally, whole grains (except wheat) help reduce fat in the body. Spinach is such a great source of iron, which is vital for our red blood cells to keep our systems going. Remember, iron helps us absorb oxygen into the bloodstream. Oxygen equals more energy. Think back on how you feel when you breathe fresh air.

1
2
3
4
5
6
7
8
9
10
11

Do

Hudry Wusch Technique:

Cook the quinoa by placing one part grain into two parts water in a pot. Bring the water to a boil, turn down the heat, and let it simmer 10 more minutes until all the water is absorbed. A rice cooker is just as fast and simple to use, with no effort as well.

Roast the onions in a frying pan and blanch the broccoli florets as explained in the recipe above. Cut the spinach and anchovies and place them in a large salad bowl.

Toss and mix the quinoa over the roasted onions, blanched broccoli, spinach that is cut into small pieces, and the anchovies. Season the salad with lemon juice and olive oil for taste. Let the salad sit for 2 to 3 minutes so that the spinach mixture warms, and then serve and enjoy.

TIP! Replace the quinoa with other grains, such as brown rice, millet, or amaranth.

ALPINE
WEIGHT LOSS
SECRETS

SESAME SEED SEARED TUNA with
TOMATOES SHIITAKE SAUCE and a SPELT BUN

Look

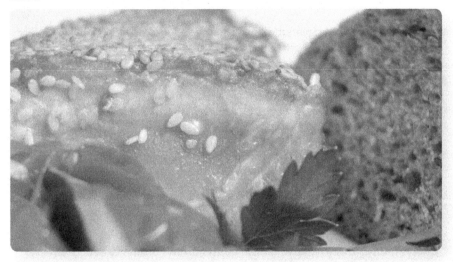

Learn

Ingredients:

1 piece wild tuna

1 pint organic baby tomatoes

3 medium-size shiitake mushrooms

3 minced garlic cloves

3 tablespoons sesame seeds

Extra virgin olive oil

Sea salt

Spelt bun

Benefits:

The omega 3 fatty acids found in fish are super workers. They support brain function and the glandular system, which drives metabolism, improves the body's immune response, and reduces the severity of migraine headaches. They also are beneficial for rheumatoid arthritis. Studies have proved that shiitake mushrooms have powerful antiviral properties, lower blood cholesterol, and enhance circulation. In other words, they have been proven to enhance and stimulate your system, in particular your immune system. Yes, there is real science behind my program.

Do

Hudry Wusch Technique:

Cut the washed baby tomatoes in half and simmer slowly in preheated olive oil in a covered sauté pan. After 5 minutes add the washed, thinly sliced shiitake mushrooms and allow to simmer for another 10 minutes until the tomatoes have turned into a sauce.

Sear the washed tuna, covered with sesame seeds, in a stir-fry pan that is slightly covered with olive oil for about 5 minutes, on each side. If you prefer it medium rare, cook for a shorter time; for well-done tuna, sear longer. Keep warm in the preheated oven at 200°F until the sauce is done.

Heat the spelt bun in the heated oven for about 3 minutes. Season the sauce with a little salt and the small chopped garlic cloves at the very end before serving. Serve, sit down, and enjoy.

TIP! This recipe serves one person, but why not double it and invite a friend to join you?

ORGANIC CURRIED EGG SALAD on WHOLE-GRAIN BREAD

Look

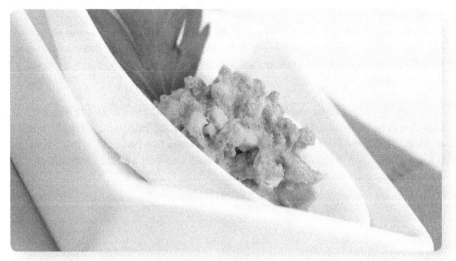

Learn

Ingredients:

5 hard-boiled organic eggs with egg yolks
½ diced red onion
2 slices whole-grain bread
1 tsp Indian curry
2 tablespoons extra virgin olive oil
Sea salt

Benefits:

Eggs have a very high Net Protein Utilization (NPU), so the body is able to use the natural protein more efficiently than that found in many other foods. Other foods high in NPU (in order of merit) are: fish, brown rice, red meat, and poultry. Did you notice eggs, fish, and brown rice come before red meat and poultry? When exercising, or during times of illness, surgery, or injury, our bodies require higher protein production to help restore the body's strength through the regeneration of cells and tissues. Of course the utilization of protein is maximized when you are working out 5 to 6 times per week.

Do

Hudry Wusch Technique:

Boil the eggs. This should not take longer than 3 minutes. Place eggs in cold water and bring to a boil. When the eggs are ready, shock them with cold water and peel them. Cut the eggs into smaller pieces and place in a medium salad bowl.

Dice the onion while boiling the eggs. Mix in the diced onion over the eggs.

Mix the olive oil, sea salt, and curry to taste, but be careful, as the curry is very, very flavorful. Serve the warm egg salad over whole-grain rye bread, and cut into small pieces.

TIP! This is very delicious. Careful that you don't eat the entire thing in 2 minutes. I have heard it has happened before. Also choose one dish from the Veggie Bonanza, and one carbohydrate from the Best category to make your meal complete. Or take it to work. Place the egg salad in the middle of a mustard green, roll and wrap. Enjoy.

VEGGIE BONANZA

Many of my clients are excited about starting to cook. Some of you are frightened but thrilled when you realize how easy it is and that many of the vegetables in my program mentioned are interchangeable within recipes. Here are some items that are simple to prepare, that you can make in less than 5 minutes. Just choose a carbohydrate and protein from the Best category and one of the below items, and your simple lunch or dinner will be ready.

CAULIFLOWER with SEASONING

Ingredients:
3 cups cauliflower florets
1 lemon, fresh-squeezed juice
¼ tsp turmeric
Extra virgin olive oil
Sea salt

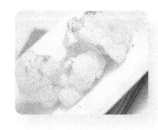

Cut cauliflower into medium-size pieces.
Blanch in boiling water for about 2 minutes, until tender.
Drain and season with olive oil, sea salt, lemon juice, and turmeric

TIP! To intensify the flavor, try placing blanched and seasoned cauliflower on a baking sheet, place in the oven for 30 to 40 minutes at 400°F, and cook until the vegetables are caramelized.

STRING BEANS with GINGER and GARLIC

Ingredients:
½ lb organic string beans
¼ tsp ground ginger
2 minced gloves of garlic
Extra virgin olive oil
Sea salt

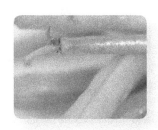

Blanch beans for 2 minutes but no longer.
Heat up an omelet pan, and add olive oil, ginger, and sliced garlic.
Toss the string beans in when the spices start to give up a delicious smell. Stir, turn the heat off, and cover for 1 to 2 minutes.

SAUTEED KALE

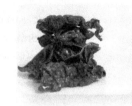

Ingredients:
1 bunch organic kale
Extra virgin olive oil
Sea salt

Wash the kale and leave dripping wet while cutting into thick strips. Remove the pieces with the thick stem.
Heat the olive oil in a pan and place the wet kale in the pan and cover. Cook for 1½ minutes, then turn the kale and reduce heat. Simmer for another 1½ minutes and turn off the heat.
Season with sea salt, and let the kale simmer for 2 to 3 minutes so it can cook in its own juice.

MUSTARD GREENS

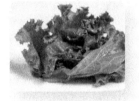

Ingredients:
1 bunch organic mustard greens
Extra virgin olive oil
Sea salt

Rinse the greens and leave dripping wet while cutting into thick strips.
Heat the olive oil in a pan and place wet greens into the pan and cover. Cook for 1½ minutes, then turn the greens and reduce the heat. Simmer for another 1½ minutes and turn off the heat.
Season with sea salt, and allow to simmer for 2 to 3 minutes so it can cook in its own juice.

SHIITAKE MUSHROOMS

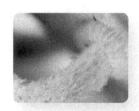

Ingredients:
5 shiitake mushrooms
1 stem fresh rosemary
Extra virgin olive oil
Sea salt

Wash the shiitake mushrooms and cut the stems into quarters.
Place the mushroom tops upside down in a baking pan covered with olive oil.
Sprinkle with a little more olive oil, sea salt, and freshly cut rosemary.
Roast in a preheated oven, 400°F, for about 20 to 30 minutes or until golden brown. Be sure not to burn the mushrooms.

PEPPER MEDLEY

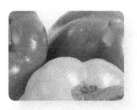

Ingredients:
5 peppers (red, green, or yellow)
3 chopped garlic cloves
Extra virgin olive oil
Sea salt

Wash the peppers and cut lengthwise into 4 even pieces. Oil the bottom of a baking pan and place the peppers in the pan, with the skin side facing up.
Roast at 400°F until the skin starts to brown, about 15 to 20 minutes. When done, remove peppers and let them cool.
Serve as they are or peel the skin, slice lengthwise, and mix in the garlic. Sprinkle with sea salt and serve.

TIP! Puree the peppers and enjoy as a spread for vegetables or rye crisps. Great for breakfast as well.

KOHLRABI

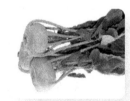

Ingredients:
3 kohlrabie
Sea salt

Peel the kohlrabi and slice thinly.
Plate it and season with sea salt. Cover with another plate, and place in refrigerator for 5 minutes, or until you're ready to serve. In Austria, we refer to this as making the vegetable sweat.
Serve as an appetizer. Your guests will be dying to know what it is.

ROASTED BEETS with GOAT CHEESE

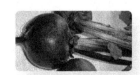

Ingredients:
1 bunch red beets
1 goat cheese
Extra virgin olive oil and sea salt

Chop off the greens and wash the roots under cold water.

Bake the roots in an olive oil-covered glass baking dish that is covered tightly (with a dish cover or aluminum foil) so that you lock in the moisture. Bake at 450°F for between 30 and 40 minutes. Allow to cool.

Slice the beets after cooling and plate them with the goat cheese cut length-wise. Sprinkle with a little olive oil and sea salt, and you are ready to eat. It's so simple and very delicious.

TIP! These veggies need very little attention. Pop them in the oven while you are busy with other things. Try roasting the beets before you leave for work in the morning. Simply turn off the oven and let them continue to cook while you are gone.

Caution! Of course, no cheese during the first 14 days. Why? Because it is processed and lacks friendly bacteria to support your digestion. Also keep in mind lactose intolerance. This is for you to find out while you go through the program. In the meantime, enjoy them just roasted, or make a beet salad with chopped onions, chopped parsley, and some olive oil and sea salt for seasoning.

HEIRLOOM TOMATOES with

BASIL and BUFFALO MOZZARELLA

Ingredients:
2 heirloom tomatoes
1 bunch basil
1 small fresh buffalo mozzarella

Stefan, this is not cooking. Yeah, so what? Who wants to cook all the time? The key is to get you thinking about how to prepare meals with the least amount of effort possible with ingredients that taste good to help you lose weight and look younger.

Wash the tomatoes and basil. Pat the basil with paper towel until dry and slice the tomatoes.

Slice the mozzarella after draining the liquid from the mozzarella.

Layer the tomato and mozzarella on one of your beautiful plates. Make it look nice! When you are done, take a few basil leaves and stick them between or around your stack.

TIP! A great, cold summer dish on a hot day when it's too hot to turn on the oven!

Caution! You guessed it: not a 14-day Alpine Eating friendly recipe...but it will be friendly without the mozzarella.

YELLOW SALAD

Ingredients:
3 organic carrots
2 organic celery sticks
½ tsp turmeric
1 tsp tahini
2 tsp extra virgin olive oil
Sea salt

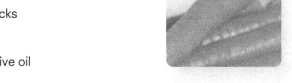

Wash the carrots and celery.
Cut them into small pieces (don't dice them) and place them in a salad bowl.
Season and mix with turmeric, two teaspoons of tahini (buy organic, in the glass and not in a can), and a dash of sea salt and olive oil. The first time I ate this, I almost wet myself it was so good...I ate the whole bowl (the salad, not the bowl itself).

RED GREEN CHUNKY SOUP

Ingredients:
4 organic tomatoes
1 cucumber
½ diced onion
1 tablespoon chopped parsley
Extra virgin olive oil
Sea salt

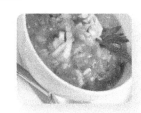

Wash and then cut the tomatoes into quarters and blend in a blender by pressing chop instead of liquid. You want this to have texture and not be a liquid. After blending the tomatoes, place the tomato mixture in a big salad bowl.
Peel and chop the cucumber into chunky pieces. Dice the onions as well and mix together.
Season with sea salt, olive oil, and chopped parsley to your liking. Decorate with parsley and serve.

TIP! If you have digestive issues, you might want to heat the soup up briefly. Or leave the cucumber out, heat the soup slowly for 20 to 25 minutes, and use it as your pasta sauce.

TABOULI SALAD

Ingredients:
4 cups quinoa
2 bunches parsley
2 white onions
1 pint organic baby tomatoes
4 lemons
Olive oil
Sea salt

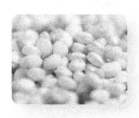

If you have been following my recipes, you will know I am a huge fan of quinoa. So what to do when you've made a big batch and have so much left over? Make tabouli salad!

Cook 2 cups of quinoa and 4 cups of water in a rice cooker. Add a little sea salt and olive oil for taste. Simmer for about 10 minutes.
Chop the parsley after washing and the onion. Squeeze the juice of 4 lemons and reserve. Cut the tomatoes into small pieces but keep them chunky. Mix all the ingredients in a large salad bowl, and, finally, pour on the lemon juice.
Season to taste with sea salt and olive oil, and serve in a small salad bowl.

TIP! It tastes best when the quinoa is a little bit warm, almost straight out of the pot.

ALPINE SURVIVAL SALAD

Ingredients:
½ bunch romaine lettuce
½ pint baby tomatoes
½ red onion
1 green bell pepper
3 tsp sunflower seeds
1 lemon, freshly squeezed juice
3 tsp extra virgin olive oil
1 pinch sea salt
1 cup leftover grain if you like (brown rice or quinoa)

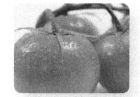

Wash all the vegetables, except the onion, then tear the romaine lettuce into small pieces and place in the salad bowl.
Cut the baby tomatoes in half, chop the onion, cut the green bell pepper lengthwise (it gets boring if everything is the same size), and toss everything on top of the lettuce. If you like, mix in your grains at this time.
Mix your dressing of olive oil, sea salt and lemon juice… toss with salad and sunflower seeds. So light and refreshing on a humid night.

RADISHES with ANCHOVY PASTE

Ingredients:
1 bunch organic radishes
½ anchovy paste tube
Extra virgin olive oil

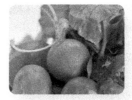

Wash the radishes.
Cut the radishes in quarters but leave the long root intact.
Mix the anchovy paste and olive oil in a bowl, place the radishes in the center, and you are ready to go. Enjoy!

TIP! To prevent bloating and gas problems, please don't eat 3 bunches of radishes at once...even if you really like it.
TIP! Be creative! Enjoy your food, and mix it up... just stay within the guidelines of the program. Remember, like any new venture... plan, organize, and execute. Practice will make your new skill set become second nature in no time.

SPREADS

Why spreads? Because they are fast and easy to make. Hudry Wusch! Besides this, some of them are great breakfast solutions, or just really nice to prepare as appetizers for your dinner parties.

CARROT ONION SPREAD

Ingredients:
20 carrots, cut and washed
3 large chopped onions
Black pepper
Extra virgin olive oil
Sea salt

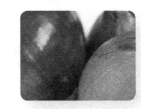

Steam the washed and cleaned carrots slowly until soft, and then let them cool off a little.
Stir-fry the onion until golden brown. Mix the onion with the carrots, and mash them all together. Imagine that you are making mashed potatoes just with carrots.
Season with sea salt and some pepper to your liking. If you like, you can add olive for additional flavor. Hey, yes, but only if you have really good, fresh-pressed olive oil. Don't settle for cheap alternatives.

TIP! Eat that spread in the morning instead of jam.

YOGURT SPREAD

Ingredients:
1 yogurt strainer
(go on the Internet to Google for one;
they are great)
1 pint of nonfat plain yogurt
1 bunch of chives or other herbs

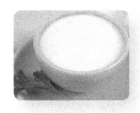

Strain the yogurt overnight.
Chop up all the herbs of your choice and mix them with the yogurt.
Serve with a little bit of sea salt or some red pepper. This is also very easy to
serve just plain as a spread, and it takes no time.

TIP! Another great breakfast spread. Tastes like cream cheese, but it is not.

BASIL SPREAD

Have you ever gone to the farmers market and bought a humungous bunch of
basil that sits rotting in your refrigerator a week later? Doesn't that drive you
crazy? Here are a couple of good solutions: Make the tomato and mozzarella
dish. Wrap the remaining basil tightly in plastic or place the stems in a glass of
water. Or make this delicious basil spread. Here goes:

Ingredients:
1 bunch fresh basil
Extra virgin olive oil
Sea salt

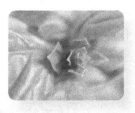

Wash and chop the basil after separating the tender
leaves and stems. Chop, chop, chop it into very small
pieces, so it almost becomes a spread by itself. Place
the chopped basil in a bowl.
Mix in olive oil and season with sea salt. Use only enough oil so it becomes a
spread.
Served best on fresh organic rye or spelt bread.

TIP! Make fresh before serving and use the following 2 days.

LIPTAUER SPREAD

Ingredients:
2 packages farmer's cheese
1 chopped hard-boiled egg
1½ diced white onions
1 tablespoon small chopped capers
1 tablespoon mustard (sugar free)
1 tsp red paprika powder
¼ tsp black pepper
Sea salt

Chop the egg, onion, and capers. Then mix and stir the farmer's cheese in a bowl until it has a smoother texture.
Mix all together and season with sea salt, mustard, paprika powder, and some black pepper to your liking. The taste is up to you. You can make the Liptauer sharper if you add more paprika or black pepper. It is really a personal preference.
Serve it with carrot or celery sticks.

TIP! It's best to prepare Liptauer a day before serving, so the flavors will be fully developed. PSSST...if you like, you can add in some finely chopped sardines as well. Not a friendly recipe for the first 14 days unless you replace the farmer's cheese with strained yogurt.

1
2
3
4
5
6
7
8
9
10
11

DESSERT

What are we going to do for some dessert solutions after your initial 14-day program? Here are my top recommendations, besides having fruits for dessert. Please, please, please call me when you make the Viennese Apple Strudel.

THE ENERGY CRUNCH

Look

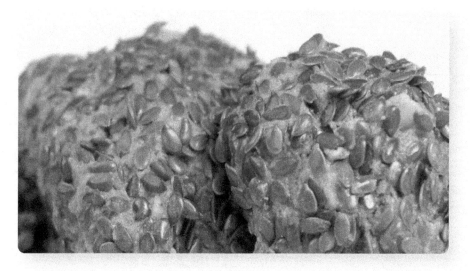

Learn

Ingredients:
1 cup barley flour or oat flour
1½ cups oat flakes or oatmeal
¾ cup almond flakes
1 tsp baking soda
2 eggs
2 tsp ground cinnamon
1 tsp allspice
1 tsp almond extract
2 tsp vanilla extract
½ cup almond butter
½ cup extra virgin olive oil (use 1 cup apple sauce instead if concerned about oil)
½ cup brown rice syrup
Flaxseeds in which to roll the Crunch

Benefits:
The Energy Crunch is great to have as a snack, with tea, for dessert, or just

because you feel like chewing on something. Most ingredients improve your health; the oats help neutralize excess cholesterol; it's chockful of calcium, iodine, phosphorus, iron, vitamin E (great for your skin); and don't forget the immune-boosting B complex. And a healthy reminder: "3 almonds a day keep the doctor away!" Almonds and almond oil are rich in vitamins A, C, E, and minerals like zinc, potassium, chromium, iron, and copper… all of which nourish your immune system. The bottom line is these nutritious cookies will satisfy your cravings while they improve your digestion, overall health, and appearance. Hey, wait; I didn't say you should live on them.

Do

Hudry Wusch Technique:

Mix all the dry ingredients. After mixing all the dry ingredients, combine the remaining wet ingredients and mix them all together. If it is too sticky, add some flour.

Form balls, approximately 2 tablespoons in size, with two tablespoons, and roll in flaxseed. Place on a nonstick baking sheet, covered with parchment paper.

Bake for 15 to 20 minutes in a preheated oven at 350°F. Make sure you don't burn them by leaving them in the oven for too long… it has happened before.

TIP! Substitute brown rice or buckwheat flour, in case you are gluten Intolerant. Leave the oats out as well and increase the almond flakes to one and one-half cups. More about gluten in the next recipe.

CATHERINE CAKE

Look

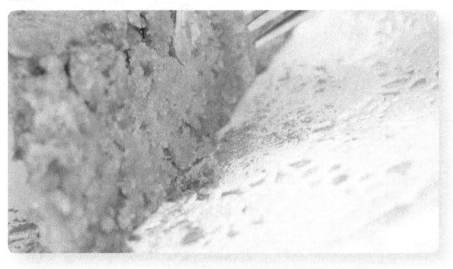

Learn

Ingredients:

2 cups spelt flour

1 cup oat flour

1 cup brown rice syrup

1 cup olive oil

1 tsp aluminum-free baking powder

2 eggs

3 cups shredded carrots

2 cups shredded zucchini

1 cup walnuts

Benefits:

Hudry Wusch, Hudry Wusch, and Hudry Wusch. I swear it is really that easy.
This was another invention of mine because I was so bored with all the buttery
and sugary desserts that don't taste like anything and don't provide nutrition.
At least when you eat dessert, eat desserts that are nutritious. You can use
other flours such as whole wheat, oat, rye, corn, barley, rice, buckwheat,
millet, amaranth, and quinoa (listed from the most common allergenic to the
least common). If you are concerned about gluten allergy, use only soy,
millet, corn, rice, quinoa, and buckwheat flour. Most importantly, notice
the fiber content in this recipe from the whole grains. This makes the

difference between a great, healthy body and poor health. Hey, I hope you have learned about fiber already! No? Then the next time I will slap your bottom as punishment if I ask you and you don't know it. (Sorry, but I grew up in the '80s in Austria. You know about the Christian schools and their bamboo sticks. So forget about the lovely Sound of Music).

Do

Hudry Wusch Technique:

Gather and prepare all the ingredients. Most of the work involved will be shredding the veggies, so start with them.

Mix both the shredded vegetables with the spelt and oat flour and the aluminum-free baking powder. Slowly fold in the eggs, followed by the brown rice syrup and olive oil. And finally, add the walnuts, which add to the crunchiness of the cake, and spread the dough in a cake pan. Don't forget to oil the pan.

Bake the cake for 45 minutes to 1 hour in a preheated oven at 350°F, until the top is golden brown. To ensure that the cake is well done, check with a toothpick after 40 minutes. If there is still dough on the toothpick after inserting it into the middle of the cake, it will need more time. This is a very moist cake, so be patient.

1
2
3
4
5
6
7
8
9
10
11

VIENNESE APPLE STRUDEL

Look

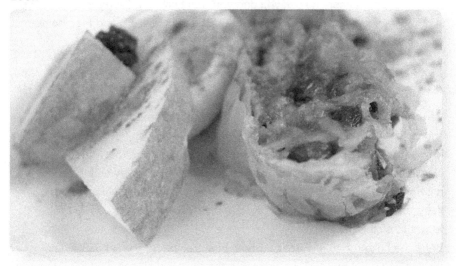

Learn

Ingredients:
5 thinly sliced apples
2 lemons, fresh-squeezed juice
1 tsp cinnamon
½ cup raisins
2 cups roasted bread crumbs (optional)
1 roll organic whole-wheat phyllo dough

Benefits:
Apples are high in fiber and have small amounts of the trace minerals that help keep your immune system strong. Fiber keeps your blood sugar and insulin levels in check. Yes, you know already when your blood sugar crashes: you become an eating machine and eat everything around you. Fiber helps you feel satisfied, and it's a satisfaction you don't get from processed snack bars. Fiber collects and holds bile acid. Yes, something has to take the garbage out of your body, and that's fiber's job. And no, don't put a dollop of whipped cream on the strudel; stay away from it.

Do

Hudry Wusch Technique:
Wash the apples and grate them in a large bowl.
Roast the breadcrumbs in olive oil until they are dark brown, and add the lemon juice, cinnamon, raisins, and roasted breadcrumbs to the grated apples.

ALPINE
WEIGHT LOSS
SECRETS

Mix them all together. Then prepare the phyllo dough on a kitchen towel and place the apple filling in a thick strip on one end of the phyllo dough. Roll the dough and ingredients together, starting from the filling to the other end, and place on a baking sheet.

Bake it for 45 minutes to 1 hour in the preheated oven of 350°F, until the top is golden brown.

TIP! This dish is a simple way to impress your family, girlfriend, or boy-friend, or even a first date. And don't forget, first impressions count.

SUCCESS!

"You need to give me recipes" many clients requested after reading the program. The recipes will get you started. Take is step by step; this is a learning experience.

The beauty about this program is that you don't have to cook. Rather you can assemble the ingredients such as given in the sample programs. Pick 3 ingredients and work with seasonings to enhance the flavor. Let the flavor from the food stimulate your taste buds instead of butter, creams, and sauces.

It is a process. Making food taste to your liking is easy. The recipes will help you to find your taste buds again with the least amount of effort. Don't get frustrated. Learning a new skill will take a little patience. After 1 week, you should be able to master it. If you are used to cooking you will have it a little easier, but it will depend on your style. The recipes teach you to work with the flavor of a chosen ingredient that is beneficial to your weight loss and to look younger naturally. Think about how long it would take you to learn a new foreign language! With effort you will find good-tasting ingredients in your area. And this would be 90% of your work in the beginning. The rest will fall into place, and it is no effort to implement. Explore and discover your neighborhood. Perhaps a new store, supermarket, or farm is waiting for you to discover and there you will find the ingredients listed in my program.

Remember, you have set your goal. Now, do anything possible to get there. Read the ingredients! Don't take it easy and be serious about what you do. Start taking responsible actions and explore what possibilities you have.

The Alpine Shopping List

Where can you buy the ingredients for the program?

Buy from your local farmers or farmer's market. Some of these farmers can be very interesting characters! In most cities, they have organized farmer's markets, where local growers come in on designated days to sell their products. This allows you to know where their items come from, how they were grown or raised, and gives you direct contact with the providers. No supermarket can tell you how the last harvest went or which cow is about to have a baby. Search online for green markets or farmers markets in your area. If you live in New York City, go to www.cenyc.org to find locations and times.

Supermarkets that focus on bringing the best foods to the consumer have been coming up and very successful in the food-provision arena. Whole Foods and Fresh Fields are 2 of the first who managed to raise the food industry standard. You will discover many hard-to-find ingredients there. You can also pick up very tasty, well-prepared food on the run from their selection of freshly prepared foods.

Health-food stores and food co-ops are another choice. Before Whole Foods and Fresh Fields came around, health food stores and food co-ops were the places to go to. There you can buy ingredients in bulk. Compare and contrast. Whole Foods has been many times called "Whole Paycheck," but when you compare the prices to a regular supermarket and health food stores, they will win straight out. In either case, if budget is a consideration, you will find the best possible solution for you after you have done your comparison research.

The Alpine Shopping List

Shopping is easy if you know what to look for. Let me help you. Find a list of ingredients on page 183 that you want to stock at home. You always can snack on them or have them ready for a meal. As a general rule, try to buy organic over conventional food.

- Vegetables listed in category 1 and 2; buy organic before you buy conventional
- Proteins such as fish, chicken, and turkey; buy wild raised, cage free, and natural feed
- Carbohydrates such as grains; buy only organic

Make it easier for you. Make a copy of the 14-day Fresh Air Foods Program and the shopping list, and go shopping with it. Choose the items that you like and know first, and work with them. Use the next shopping trip to discover a new ingredient. Make it work for you.

Food Item	Item Description	Company / Brand
Salad	Baby Arugula Salad Baby Lettuce Mixed Bay Greens Fresh Herb Salad	Earth Bound Farm
Hummus	All Natural Hummus All Natural with Roasted Garlic All Natural Traditional Style	Abraham's
Mochi	Sesame Garlic Original	Grainnaissance
Olive Oil	Olio Verde Capezzana	Manicaretti
Dressing	Shiitake & Sesame Vinaigrette	Annie's Natural
Pasta	Vita Spelt Whole Wheat Rice Pasta	Purity Foods Westbrae & Natural De Boles
Flour	Spelt Oat Rye	Arrowhead Mills
Fish	Anchovy Fillets	Manicaretti
Crackers	Baked Woven Wheats	365 Whole Foods
Tea	Peppermint Tea Chamomile	Celestial Seasoning
Butters	Almond	Maranatha
Jams	Black Raspberry Wild Blueberry Red Raspberry	St. Dalfour
Turkey	Turkey Burger	Applegate Farms
Yogurt	Plain Nonfat Low-fat	Stony Fields Horizon
Eggs	Local/Cage Free (best)	Their are many
Bread	Spelt Bread Hearty Rye	The Baker Wasa
Cereal	Original	Ezekiel 4:6
Milk	Rice Dream /Original	Rice Dream
Juice	Unsweetened Cranberry Juice	Knudson

9 Steps to Success

❶ **Learn.** Read and familiarize yourself with the Fresh Air Foods Program.

❷ **Prepare.** Buy the necessary ingredients and stock up your pantry.

❸ **Discover.** Find restaurants or stores where you can eat on the run.

❹ **Structure.** Get organized and understand what you are about to do.

❺ **Start.** Set a date, get started, and stay focused on your goal.

❻ **Taste.** Buy good olive oil. When you cook and season your food with disgusting tasting olive oil, you won't eat it. Even if the food is organic. Manicaretti offers the best tasting oil. And my clients agree.

❼ **Simple.** Stay simple first. Boil eggs to have them ready at hand. Salad with 3 other ingredients would be next. It doesn't take effort to wash the ingredients, toss them together, and season them for a simple main meal.

❽ **Seasoning.** Lemon is the key. Season your food for one week with lemon. Stay away from creams or other dressing. Discover the lemon, sea salt, and olive oil flavor. You will be hooked after 1 day.

❾ **Succeed.** Make it work for you. This will become your program, not mine!

Chapter 11

"HOLODRIO!" STAY, FEEL, AND LOOK YOUNG FOR A LIFETIME

Holodrio! What does it mean?

When you go on a hiking trip and you climb over the last ledge to the peak, see the sunrays reflect on the clouds that flood below you, while feeling rejuvenated and energized, and this warm fuzzy feeling takes over you, then you know you reached out and accomplished what you set out to do. This moment is expressed as Holodrio. Everything came together. You did it.

Even if you don't live in an Alpine environment, you can apply my Alpine mindset anywhere (as so many of our clients have done in New York City). The key is to make them work for you and your lifestyle. Is it tough sometimes? Sure, but we have the mental tips to keep you motivated. Is it worth the effort? Just look in the mirror! Bask in the compliments: "You look great! Was it a new dermatologist or surgery?" Neither. It was all due to the transformative power of fresh-air foods and fitness!

Basics Revisited

Let's revisit the basic principles of the program:

- Change your mind to change your body; and keep a food log and flex your mental muscle.

- Think about light when it comes to eating your fruits and vegetables.

- Buy at the farmer's market instead of in the supermarket.

- Eat with each meal 1 portion of foods that are raw foods (salad first) to provide your body enzymes for a functioning metabolism.

- Eat from your gut and not from a brain full of nuts.

- Make better decisions when ordering your meals.

- Eat greens over grains during your weight loss.

- Use lime and lemon for seasoning and flavoring of your food.

- Drink up. Drink lemon or lime-flavored (fresh only) water during the program.

- Manage your insulin levels and stay off and away from sugars (including fruit sugar for 14 days).

- Add avocado, nuts, seeds, olive oil, and pumpkin oil to your salads. Raw fats help to burn fat (biological fats only).

- Ground flaxseeds go well with your breakfast or over salads.

- Eat beets to cleanse your liver for your fat metabolism.

- Repair your DNA with sardines.

- Improve your posture and think Alignment, Activation, and Elongation.

- Discover your inner child and have fun with the activities you enjoy.

- Breathe fresh air for stress management and celebrate yourself with each single step you take while enjoying the outdoors.

- Think and be thin. Build up your Mountain Program to twice a week.

- Juice it up to flatten your belly or start with the 2-Day Alpine Cleansing Cure kick-start program.

- Be honest, check in with yourself to find yourself and ensure your direction.

- Explore and discover 2 new ingredients per week.

- Assemble foods into a 5-star dining experience with the Hudry Wusch technique.

- Ask the right questions to avoid getting stuck and move forward in your transformation process.

- Men need more calories than women (1,800 vs. 1,200).

- Vary your program with the Mountain, Hill, and Valley programs.

- Change it up with rest, repetitions, resistance, set, and speed.

- Learn the Alpine Longevity Strength Moves and build up to the shortcut program with the Alpine Youngevity Fitness Program.

Changes will happen. And they will happen when you change your mind to change your body when flexing your mental muscle. Flexing your mental muscle is a radical change in your behavior. Yes, this is your objective—change step by step from one day to the next. To help you along the way and give you inspiration as to how clients have managed their changes, let me introduce you to Margarita, Vikki, and Casey.

Case Studies: Margarita, Vikki, and Casey

Margarita, 55 years old

Margarita, 55, gained weight after each of her 3 children. Finally her doctor told her that to avoid a quadruple by-pass surgery, she needed to lose weight. At 5 feet 2 inches and 220 pounds, she fell in the obese category. The meniscus operation on each leg set her back one more time.

On the initial consultation, we determined her goal. She knew that she couldn't have a model figure, but she wanted to look the best for her body shape. Weight loss, toning, and shaping were her goal while improving her health. When meeting her, it was clear that she did belong in another body. She walked slowly, shifted her weight from side to side, and seemed to be a little disoriented. Yet she was quick to understand the information provided. Although she was working out regularly (light weights and walking), she had managed to lose weight and regain it. This was her first attempt to work with a personal coach to lose the weight and keep it off to prevent her heart surgery.

We agreed to keep a food log. My first glance at her food log set the program for her. Margarita is of Dominican heritage, and her habits have been influenced by it. Her diet consisted of fried food, rice and beans, yucca, cereal, fried banana, and all cooked foods. After pointing out the starchy carbohydrates over the fibrous carbohydrates, she saw that her diet was dominated by starchy carbohydrates. The colors green, orange, and yellow were missing. Fats came from frying oils. And there were great items on her food log as well, such as salmon, eggs, yogurt, and lime juice.

Colors were the secret to her success. To make her realize how out of balance her diet was, we used 3 colors to create an "Aha" effect. I used the colors brown for starchy carbohydrates, green for fibrous carbohydrates, and pink for protein. This task revealed that on 1 page of her log only 3 circles of green appeared after 5 days of eating.

My goal was clear in her progress. First, I was to explain to her the importance of enzymes in her diet, the function of enzymes, and how enzymes were killed through cooking. My number 1 advice to her was to increase her greens and my number 2 advice was to increase her enzymes in her diet.

Breakfast was the start of her downfall. Her day started with a large cereal bowl with milk and a French vanilla coffee. After explaining to her the importance of maintaining insulin levels during a weight loss program, we started changing her breakfast to oatmeal with cinnamon and hot tea. My advice was to drink a full glass of water and the freshly squeezed juice of half a lemon first thing in the morning (the Alpine Eye-Opener).

One week showed the difference in her body. From one week to the next her energy improved. She moved quicker and did not feel sleepy during the day. She reported that she started to feel lighter when she ate more greens. Cucumber slices with a little salt and lemon was her preferred snack instead of juice and coffee. Step by step she adjusted to the eating plan.

Joy in her exercise program came when she changed her cardio intensity. As a regular exerciser, she knew the benefits of exercise. But by doing the same thing over again, she hit a plateau, and the results stayed the same. Next, my goal was to educate her toward a program that burned the most calories of fat in a short time. The Mountain Program was implemented after we established reference points of comfort levels for how much she could push herself. My advice was to speed up to a point where she got out of breath and slow down to recover again. After 3 weeks she reported that walking the stairs became easier, and her legs kept up with the endurance program.

Working with heavier weight toned her body. She was used to working with only light resistance. After years lifting weights, her body shape stayed the same without any change. During this phase of the program my strategy was to build up lean muscle weight by increasing the resistance. Instead of working with 5-pound hand weights, we increased to 8 pounds, 10 pounds, and to 15 pounds.

The measurements showed the results. After 4 weeks, we took measurements again. The results were not just stunning, they were excellent. Without a struggle to implement the diet changes, and using the Mountain Program and the increased resistance, she went from 221 to 210 pounds, her waist measurement from 55 inches to 44 inches, and her body fat from 39% to 37%. A total loss of 11 pounds, 2% body fat, and 20.5 inches in total circumference (12 weeks later she accomplished a weight loss of 42 pounds). Do her little changes in eating and activity seem like deprivation or torture to you?

Vikki, 41 years old

Vikki was soon to be 41 years old and had struggled with her weight her entire life, including battling several eating disorders, which she eventually overcame but with significant weight gains. Like a fashion victim who doesn't know how to dress because she was never taught what works and why, Vikki was a nutrition victim. She never learned what to eat and why. Her weight had risen and fallen by 30 to 60 pounds frequently for almost 20 years.

Besides being a perpetual binge eater and eating for comfort, she led a stress-filled life, balancing a hectic career with family responsibilities. On top of it, she had suffered a battery of health problems from multiple miscarriages to pre-diabetes and a heart condition—all within the past 6 years. Every time she lost a few pounds, something would happen and she would just fall off the wagon and the cycle continued. Diets through her life were her downfall, but she had some success with Nutrisystem, which taught her portion control. But when she left the program, she gained back all 50 pounds she had lost because she still didn't know how to eat.

First, after she started the Alpine Weight Loss Program, a different reaction took her by surprise. She said straight out that the first week was hell as she adjusted to eating only foods that supported her system. She learned that sugar and caffeine are addictive and that it is a challenge to avoid them at first. Yet the less caffeine and processed sugar she had, the easier it became. However, it took her about 7 days to adjust. She reported that by the end of the first week her experience was aching bones, which is a sign of adjustments, cleansing, and rejuvenation of her systems.

Exhaustion was her experience as her body started to heal and her systems to clean. She slept like a bear in hibernation. Nevertheless, by the second week, everything was much better, and all her negative thoughts ("this is really hard") slowly transformed into thoughts of "I can do this."

Education and eating were her keys to success. Educating her to a solid understanding of how food actually works with her body was a refreshing approach to her instead of eating prepackaged diet food from a program that just "taught" her portion control not healthy eating habits. My advice to her on my program was, "You must eat." Too many women starve themselves on food that does not have nutritional value for the system, which therefore leaves them longing for much more. It is a vicious cycle that leads them to eat the wrong things repeatedly.

The taste was as shocking at first as the flavor was new to her. She tried the recipes and loved them. Can a recipe of such simplicity, such as the Turkey Burgers, Alpine Survival Salad, or Roasted Beets, taste so good AND keep her satisfied MUCH longer? Yes, it was possible. Hudry Wusch taught her that it is not about cooking but about assembling the right flavor combinations. As soon she followed the first recipes, she understood what she was missing in packaged food—the flavor of real nutrition.

Portion control came naturally therefore. She ate from the first 2 categories only, and surprisingly, wasn't as hungry as she once was, so she stopped eating when she was full. She remained full longer, she didn't count calories, and she didn't measure a whole lot. I advised her to eat only week 1 and week 2 menues. Now it is easier for her to just do it.

At one point she started to pay attention to how much food she ate. As an experienced dieter, she knew how to count calories. She was worried as she discovered that she had days when she ate about 1,000 calories instead of the recommended 1,200 calories (number dependant on your situation). Many experts or weight loss Web sites recommend that during a weight loss phase women should not be eating less then 1,200 calories. Yet what is overlooked is that the human body is not a machine and responds to natural calorie needs if the body is trained to listen to it. Vikki learned that over 2 weeks and stopped eating when she was full. As she had excessive energy stored around her midsection, and the liver has up to 20 days' worth of glucose stored for energy, I wasn't concerned about this occurrence. Rather, I was pleased and encouraged her to keep listening to her body. This is the zigzag approach I mentioned earlier. When you are more active, you will need a little bit more, and if less, you will need less. Your body will not go into starvation mode in 2 days while you're eating 3 regular meals and 2 snacks.

Calories where not the challenge for Vikki; it was her husband and daughter who wanted her to go back to Nutrisystem as it was "easier" for them. It was a struggle until we had a conversation about to whom she was listening. The expert or the non-experts who had an opinion? This committed her to continue to implement changes her way.

In the middle of her third week she had lost 11 pounds. She was exercising more often and had implemented the short-cut program at home. She started drinking lots of water in the morning and before lunch and dinner. Now she feels an incredible sense of control because she believes she can, for the first time in her life, tackle her weight and health issues. And this is priceless.

Learning and improving gave her the determination to stick with it. The more things she learned, the more she built up an arsenal that allowed her to stay with it. Investing more in her made her happier, less nervous, and less sweaty. (Yes, sweaty! She is perimenopausal and cutting out caffeine has made a HUGE difference.) It also helped her be less emotional, as she wrote me in an e-mail.

"You can do it" were always my encouraging words. And she did it. Today she thanks me for getting rid of all the fat, the low energy, and an old body. Her body changed, and she felt motivated to continue on the program. The last time, 5 weeks after I heard from her, she had lost 20 pounds, and I am convinced that I will receive an e-mail from her that she has lost all the 50 pounds she wanted to lose (at 12 weeks, she'd lost 30 pounds).

Casey, 62 years old

There is nothing unusual about wanting to look your best. But the main pressure comes from the external environment such as your work, your friends, or your family. Many times youth is celebrated and old age is looked at as if it was a disease. And walking like an old person, taking small steps, and a hunched-over posture doesn't help your case in a competitive, challenging market environment.

When I first meet her, Casey was great looking with great posture, a toned body, and no sign of slowing down. She was a familiar face in the neighborhood and known for staying committed to her goals. With her exercise program, she wasn't that different. Anyone who met Casey would have agreed that she was the picture of health and was perfect for her job as a social worker.

The situation changed because of a back injury. Afterward she was very hesitant to do any exercise program besides stretching and cardio training on the equipment. She only pushed herself just to a point where she felt comfortable. Also, because of her back injury, she had gained 15 pounds and lost strength and body tone. She saw me training other clients and after months of watching, reading my weekly newsletters, and reading in national magazines about my programs, she felt comfortable to hire me.

Determining her current problems was easy. A questionnaire, the body measurements, and the body analysis gave me insight into her current situation. Her body was flexible, but she did not have mid-body strength. When I first met Casey, she was one of the strongest in my classes. Motivated, always upfront, and pushing her energy systems (aerobic and anaerobic) to the max. That was at age 54. She had grace when she walked, strength, and balance wasn't a problem.

She wanted to rehabilitate after her surgery, but she also wanted to protect her back. She stopped strength training and taking classes. Her food log revealed a diet that was full of nuts, seeds, fruits, and vegetables. One needn't be an expert to see that she was afraid to move for fear she'd hurt her back again. While her food intake was healthy, it was too much for her activity level.

The first step was to strengthen her midsection to protect her back but also to provide as stable an environment as possible when she started to do functional movements again, such as the Alpine Longevity Strength Program that uses her own body weight. At the same time her overall muscular system needed to be strengthened through basic movements with her body weight again. Instead of working with machines, she needed to work in an unstable environment to not just condition the large muscle groups but all the small muscle groups that provide stability for the larger muscles. I explained to her the activation of the abdominal wall, pelvic girdle, and how she simply could work on this during the day while sitting or walking. The transverse abdominals string was a great help in accomplishing this and she started to flatten her belly though this activation.

As her goal was to flatten her stomach, she implemented the 2-day

A *Flat Belly – "Schnell" (fast)!* Program. The results were outstanding. During the aging process, digestion slows down and vitamins and minerals are not efficiently broken down as in younger years. Less secretion of gastric juices such as hydrochloric acid can cause this. A simple strategy to increase hydrochloric acid is to add fresh lemon juice to your diet. After 2 days on the Alpine Eating Program, her energy improved. After 1 week, her fat loss accelerated and her body shape changed.

The *2-day A Flat Belly – "Schnell" (fast)!* helped her to analyze her relationship with food. She knew that the quality of food is important. Hence, eating fresh and local foods wasn't new to her. Nuts and seeds were her downfall. Nuts and seeds are great fats, and you should eat them—just not in excessive quantities. We all have foods that we indulge in from time to time. When you indulge every day, it becomes an addiction. The 2-day Alpine Cleansing Cure juicing program will help you reorder your relationship to food to start with a fresh slate.

"Greens over grains" was one of the main adjustments in her eating. I also advised her to increase her protein intake because protein does not raise blood sugar levels as carbohydrates do. We needed to reduce the amount of nuts and seed she ate and replace them with better snack alternatives. In her case, it helped to drink water when she was hungry. And her nuts were counted from then on. Hard-boiled eggs, yogurt, grapefruit, and thinly sliced turkey were on her new snack list.

The mental adjustment of her relationship to food showed the results. After 4 weeks she had lost 10 pounds. Her body fat went from 32.10% to 29%. Following the Alpine Longevity Strength Program for 8 weeks and teaching her the execution of the pelvic floor, her movements and strength improved to the level she had 20 years ago. Standing on one leg became easy. Squatting to pull the beets was not an effort. Her balance and flexibility improved tremendously. She felt comfortable power-walking again as her balance and coordination improved. When her endurance improved, we gradually increased the resistance and reduced the resting periods in the program.

She found it easier to walk up stairs and keep up with daily chores. And she did not have the urge to protect her back constantly because she felt comfortable activating her abdominals and executing movements that didn't cause her pain. From one day to the next, she felt comfortable wearing a short T-shirt as her arms started to gain body tone again.

Now at age 63, she is stronger, has more endurance and better coordination than she did at age 51. Her diet has improved her current lifestyle. Instead of consuming larger portions, she has smaller portions throughout the day. Her main nutritional adjustment was to have something uncooked with every meal to improve her enzymes and not tax her system.

Margarita, Vikki, and Casey started the program with different goals. Each of them had very different issues related to health, appearance, and staying in shape. But with the science of food and exercise, they adjusted their diet and activities to their personal needs. The result was looking, feeling, and moving younger. Like many people, they assumed that at their stage of life, improvement was hopeless. Yet all their fears and concerns about pain during the aging process were irrelevant.

What does all this have to do with looking younger naturally? Everything. My advice could have been to just eat less and not worry about what you are eating. Or just start lifting weights without the proper activation of the midsection to create stability for movements to come. Or I could have not explained the science behind burning the highest amount of fat calories with the Mountain Program. Through this book I have made the point that your appearance is affected by the cellular functions of your body. Also how activities and diet stimulate your systems to keep your muscular, skeleton, cardiovascular, central nervous, endocrine, digestive, and integumentary systems in shape.

Live Younger Longer

In chapter after chapter, I have worked hard to emphasize that science is behind the advice that you will find in this book; it's mixed with experience and knowledge of what keeps many looking, feeling, and moving younger.

Why should we just dream about a 100-year-old healthy, strong, and youthful body? It is already possible to transform an older body into a younger one.

On Oprah, a 50-year-old individual was interviewed. Using diet alone, this individual transformed his heart into that of a 20-year-old with a calorie restriction diet. Is this something you should be doing? Or is this just another gimmick that is arriving on the scene?

Calorie restriction diets have been shown to slow aging. Diets that are calorie restricted slow down your metabolism, as the calorie consumption is reduced 30% to 50% below your BMR (basal metabolic requirements). Reducing calorie intake slows other systems as well (e.g., digestive enzyme production), which is believed to prolong our lifespan. Individuals who follow a calorie restriction diet consume less then 1,000 calories per day **(www.crsociety.org)**.

Optimal nutrition is required to maintain good health. But as calories are reduced, every bite counts even more, and each calorie needs to be very thoughtfully considered. You do not give any room for "off-track" behavior as this might cause malnutrition. And in today's environment, optimal nutrition means only organic foods and not conventional.

Keep in mind that you might lose more than you gain. When you exercise daily, you burn additional calories. Depending on intensity, duration, and your choice of activity, you can burn between 300 and 600 calories per hour. Your body develops lean muscle tissue that needs to be fed and maintained with additional calories. The benefit of strength training and cardiovascular training is that it not only improves your digestive, immune, skeletal, and circulatory

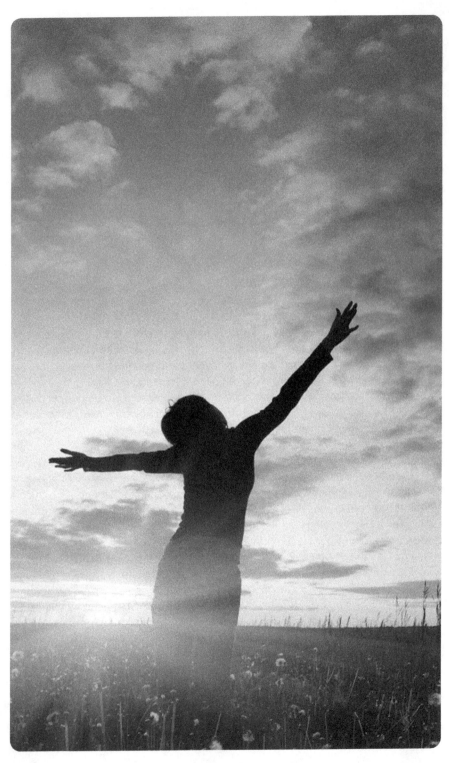

ALPINE
WEIGHT LOSS
SECRETS

systems, it has also been shown to improve mental outlook and help in managing depression.

In order to maintain an active lifestyle, you have to eat, and 1,000 calories will not be enough. If you want to gain lean muscle tissue and maintain it, you need adequate calories. Large-framed and very active individuals need more than 1,000 calories per day. A healthy, active 6-foot-tall male needs approximately 1,800 calories and a female approximately 1,200 calories. Your frame adapts to your calorie intake. Hence, when you reduce your calories below 1,000 calories, your body becomes slender. Yet when your goal is to strengthen, build muscle, and improve physical performance, calorie restriction is not beneficial, and it will work to counter your goal of building lean, fat-burning muscle tissue.

The benefits that you gain from an active lifestyle as outlined in this book are more than just a few additional years. One of the benefits of regular exercise is that you can eat and enjoy meals that have more calories because you burn them off quickly. Discovering new worlds of strength, movement, and activity improves your overall life experience and perspective. We are designed to move, not to be inactive. Our life-maintaining systems are strengthened through activity and challenged through external stress factors.

If you are planning to go on a calorie restriction diet, you need to weigh the benefit of maintaining an active lifestyle that includes regular exercise such as weightlifting, playing sports, and outdoors activities such as hiking and swimming. And an active, leaner, and strong body looks younger than a body that is not taken care of.

From my professional view, a calorie reduction diet below your BMR can be implemented at the right time with the right goal and time frame. But it may not be in your best interests when your goal is to build up lean muscle, increase performance, and to tone and shape your body as many individuals in Alpine environments do with food and activity in their natural environments.

As you can see, using **Alpine Weight Loss Secrets** to look younger naturally is just the beginning of your journey to lose weight and to look younger. Today's top scientists are discovering new ingredients or methods that slow down aging. Yet all agree that proper food and exercise will give you the best advantage in accomplishing this. Scientists also agree that the best formula for weight loss is to create a calorie deficit, which can be accomplished by increasing activity, eating less, or both. Antioxidants, flavonoids, vitamins, and minerals are other ingredients that give you the weight loss, disease prevention, and anti-aging advantage.

There is a lot to cover, and I tried to introduce you to important parts that will greatly improve the way you look, feel, and move no matter how old you are. How can I be so sure? I have seen individuals change before my eyes. It's not just their weight, body fat percentage, circumferences, energy, and attitude—lives have been changed and new directions in life have been discovered. Each triumph brings us closer to the reality of youth in older age, a slender, lean body no matter what age, and living a good life, in perfect health, to 100 years becomes a realistic and attainable goal.

ALPINE
WEIGHT LOSS
SECRETS

Additional Products and Services

What is the #1 reason that people fail to see results on a weight loss or shape up program?

Lack of motivation and support. After more than 17 years in the health, fitness, and weight loss arena, I was looking for an efficient and effective way to help people successfully stay on a program and see the results they wanted.

The most important factor that I found was to have a qualified support system, one that you can trust, one that motivates you to keep going when it gets tough, and one that pushes you when you don't want to continue.

That's why I created the **Stefan Aschan: Alpine Weight Loss Inner Circle Coaching Program**. This program is the next step in your journey to change, to stay on track, and to implement what you have learned. I will support you throughout your body makeover. I know that a one-size approach doesn't fit all. My program is all about getting the solutions that work for you.

When you participate in the **Stefan Aschan: Alpine Weight Loss Inner Circle Coaching Program**, you will receive educational online newsletters, motivational personal videos, as well as life coaching telephone sessions at different stages in the program where you can ask me any questions. This will ensure that you move forward with the right speed and progress to success! **Test it with your special trial offer.**

Access Stefan's special book purchase offer at
http://www.AlpineWeightLossSecrets.com/InnerCircleThankYou.html

Alpine Weight Loss Trips. Sign up for a week-long camp. The camps will offer you accommodation, lots of fun activities, hands-on educational seminars, and plenty of free time. Connect with like-minded people and achieve your next personal best. Those trips will be organized in the United States and Europe. Can 30 pounds be lost in 12 weeks? Yes, I have helped many of my clients to do just that. Let me share my secrets with you. Go to www.AlpineWeightLossSecrets.com/blog/alpine-weight-loss-retreat-and-seminars/ and sign up for upcoming events.

Longevity Strength Program DVD's. Work out with me. I created 3 workouts that follow the program outlined in the book. Watch as I execute the exercises with the correct form, speed and alignment. And yes, I will be yodeling here and there to make you laugh at the same time! Normally I sell those 3 DVD's individually. But I thought, why not combine them all on 1 DVD so you get three workouts for the price of one? That's just what I have done. To get your copy go to www.AlpineWeightLossSecrets.com/blog/dvd/. See the sample of the programs there as well.

Stay updated and informed. To receive your free weight loss newsletters and updates, go to www.StefanAschan.com

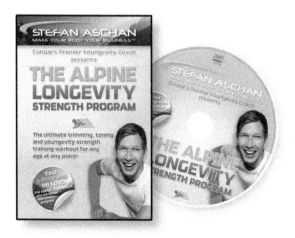

Stefan Aschan

Speaker – Author – Trainer

Stefan Aschan is one of the most professional and innovative speakers who delivers information that will make a lasting impact on your life and health.

Many companies have hired him to educate, entertain, and break up their long, monotonous training seminars (business leader seminars). Get your employees excited to work for you and show them that you care about their well-being. Cutting down on the health care costs starts with informing employees about healthy lifestyle choices, and Stefan is uniquely qualified to teach the steps to regaining and maintaining health. He addresses hundreds of people each year.

His topics include:

- Alpine stress management techniques for better health.

- When to eat this and not that.

- Seven techniques for a naturally younger you.

- What the heck is the mid-body really, and what does it have to do with me?

- How to use a string to strengthen your abs throughout the day.

- How to execute exercises to avoid injury.

Other options are available on request.

Go to **www.StefanAschan.com/ContactUs**

ALPINE
WEIGHT LOSS
SECRETS

About the Author

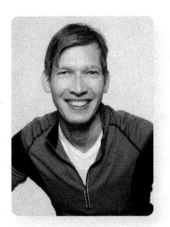

Live a healthier, trimmer, more youthful, and ener-getic life—STARTING TODAY—is Stefan Aschan's philosophy. Alpine Weight Loss Secrets explains Stefan's program that he has perfected and im-plemented for years. It incorporates his unique blend of traditional Alpine remedies and modern, cutting-edge approaches to health, fitness, gourmet cooking, and holistic nutrition. This program has helped hundreds of Stefan's clients achieve their goals.

Over the last 15 years, Stefan creatively combined his fitness, nutrition, and business training to become a leading innovator in the personal fitness, nutrition, and youngevity field. On his popular blog, www.Strength123.com, he reports on research and strategies for staying motivated, weight loss, look-ing younger longer, and staying healthy in the second half of your life. Stefan's approach to healthy living has been shaped by his Alpine upbringing, where many of his fellow villagers in their 90s are in fantastic health and living independently. Today, he regularly shares the lifestyle, weight loss, and youngevity strategies he learned in Europe and the United States with his very busy, successful, and slender clients.

As "Living" contributor to the Huffington Post, the CW11 Morning Show, and the health page of ABC News Now, Stefan is uniquely qualified to help you achieve a healthier lifestyle. In Alpine Weight Loss Secrets, he reveals strategies to achieve a healthy lifestyle and body, increase strength, and prolong youth as so many Alpine people in their 40s, 50s, and even their 90s have.

CPSIA information can be obtained
at www.ICGtesting.com
Printed in the USA
BVHW050117080223
658118BV00012B/349